T0281477

SpringerBriefs in Statistics

JSS Research Series in Statistics

Editors-in-Chief

Naoto Kunitomo, Graduate School of Economics, Meiji University, Bunkyo-ku,
Tokyo, Japan
Akimichi Takemura, The Center for Data Science Education and Research,
Shiga University, Bunkyo-ku, Tokyo, Japan

Series Editors

Genshiro Kitagawa, Meiji Institute for Advanced Study of Mathematical Sciences,
Nakano-ku, Tokyo, Japan
Tomoyuki Higuchi, The Institute of Statistical Mathematics, Tachikawa, Tokyo,
Japan
Toshimitsu Hamasaki, Office of Biostatistics and Data Mg, National Cerebral
and Cardiovascular Center, Suita, Osaka, Japan
Shigeyuki Matsui, Graduate School of Medicine, Nagoya University, Nagoya,
Aichi, Japan
Manabu Iwasaki, School of Data Science, Yokohama City University, Yokohama,
Tokyo, Japan
Yasuhiro Omori, Graduate School of Economics, The University of Tokyo,
Bunkyo-ku, Tokyo, Japan
Masafumi Akahira, Institute of Mathematics, University of Tsukuba, Tsukuba,
Ibaraki, Japan
Takahiro Hoshino, Department of Economics, Keio University, Tokyo, Japan
Masanobu Taniguchi, Department of Mathematical Sciences/School,
Waseda University/Science & Engineering, Shinjuku-ku, Japan

The current research of statistics in Japan has expanded in several directions in line with recent trends in academic activities in the area of statistics and statistical sciences over the globe. The core of these research activities in statistics in Japan has been the Japan Statistical Society (JSS). This society, the oldest and largest academic organization for statistics in Japan, was founded in 1931 by a handful of pioneer statisticians and economists and now has a history of about 80 years. Many distinguished scholars have been members, including the influential statistician Hirotugu Akaike, who was a past president of JSS, and the notable mathematician Kiyosi Itô, who was an earlier member of the Institute of Statistical Mathematics (ISM), which has been a closely related organization since the establishment of ISM. The society has two academic journals: the Journal of the Japan Statistical Society (English Series) and the Journal of the Japan Statistical Society (Japanese Series). The membership of JSS consists of researchers, teachers, and professional statisticians in many different fields including mathematics, statistics, engineering, medical sciences, government statistics, economics, business, psychology, education, and many other natural, biological, and social sciences. The JSS Series of Statistics aims to publish recent results of current research activities in the areas of statistics and statistical sciences in Japan that otherwise would not be available in English; they are complementary to the two JSS academic journals, both English and Japanese. Because the scope of a research paper in academic journals inevitably has become narrowly focused and condensed in recent years, this series is intended to fill the gap between academic research activities and the form of a single academic paper. The series will be of great interest to a wide audience of researchers, teachers, professional statisticians, and graduate students in many countries who are interested in statistics and statistical sciences, in statistical theory, and in various areas of statistical applications.

More information about this series at http://www.springer.com/series/13497

Takeshi Emura · Shigeyuki Matsui ·
Virginie Rondeau

Survival Analysis
with Correlated Endpoints

Joint Frailty-Copula Models

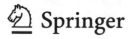 Springer

Takeshi Emura
Graduate Institute of Statistics
National Central University
Taoyuan City, Taiwan

Shigeyuki Matsui
Department of Biostatistics
Graduate School of Medicine
Nagoya University
Nagoya, Aichi, Japan

Virginie Rondeau
INSERM CR1219 (Biostatistic)
University of Bordeaux
Bordeaux Cedex, France

ISSN 2191-544X   ISSN 2191-5458   (electronic)
SpringerBriefs in Statistics
ISSN 2364-0057   ISSN 2364-0065   (electronic)
JSS Research Series in Statistics
ISBN 978-981-13-3515-0   ISBN 978-981-13-3516-7   (eBook)
https://doi.org/10.1007/978-981-13-3516-7

Library of Congress Control Number: 2019931819

© The Author(s), under exclusive license to Springer Nature Singapore Pte Ltd. 2019
This work is subject to copyright. All rights are solely and exclusively licensed by the Publisher, whether the whole or part of the material is concerned, specifically the rights of translation, reprinting, reuse of illustrations, recitation, broadcasting, reproduction on microfilms or in any other physical way, and transmission or information storage and retrieval, electronic adaptation, computer software, or by similar or dissimilar methodology now known or hereafter developed.
The use of general descriptive names, registered names, trademarks, service marks, etc. in this publication does not imply, even in the absence of a specific statement, that such names are exempt from the relevant protective laws and regulations and therefore free for general use.
The publisher, the authors and the editors are safe to assume that the advice and information in this book are believed to be true and accurate at the date of publication. Neither the publisher nor the authors or the editors give a warranty, express or implied, with respect to the material contained herein or for any errors or omissions that may have been made. The publisher remains neutral with regard to jurisdictional claims in published maps and institutional affiliations.

This Springer imprint is published by the registered company Springer Nature Singapore Pte Ltd.
The registered company address is: 152 Beach Road, #21-01/04 Gateway East, Singapore 189721, Singapore

Preface

Typical cancer clinical trials evaluate at least two survival endpoints for patients. For instance, a trial may adopt *overall survival* (OS) as the primary endpoint and *time-to-tumour progression* (TTP) as the secondary endpoint.[1] Often, the major goal of a cancer clinical trial is to estimate the effect of treatments or prognostic factors on either one or both of the endpoints. Nowadays, many databases for cancers offer individual patient data containing at least two endpoints and a number of prognostic factors (gene expressions, age, residual tumour, cancer stage, etc.).

In many cancers, the two endpoints can be strongly correlated. Indeed, one endpoint may be a *surrogate endpoint* of the other endpoint. This implies the need for an appropriate statistical model for dependence between event times. However, the standard tools, such as Cox regression, are not suitable to analyze two event times simultaneously, especially due to *dependent censoring*. For instance, early death can censor the occurrence of tumour progression. In this case, one cannot regard death as an independent censoring event from a progression event. Inappropriate account for the effect of dependent censoring may produce biased results in Cox regression.

It is even more challenging to analyze survival data when patients are collected from multiple studies (*meta-analysis* or multicenter analysis) and patients have a large number of prognostic factors. Researchers may need an advanced statistical method to characterize heterogeneity across multiple studies and to perform a feature selection tool. In the analysis of such complex survival data, it is insufficient to apply the traditional Cox regression that can only deal with a single event, a single study, independent censoring, and a small number of prognostic factors.

The book provides advanced statistical models that incorporate heterogeneity of a population in terms of frailty and dependence between endpoints in terms of copulas. Our aim is to analyze two endpoints simultaneously, where one event time is called *terminal event time* (e.g., OS) and the other event time is called *nonterminal event time* (e.g., TTP). Our main statistical tool is the *joint frailty-copula*

---

[1]Disease-free survival (DFS) and progression-free survival (PFS) are other frequently used endpoints in practice. More details about DFS, PFS, and TTP shall be discussed in Chap. 2.

model that is particularly useful for analyzing two event times simultaneously using meta-analytic data.

We focus on the pair (OS, TTP) because it is perhaps the most reasonable example to explain why the joint is useful for correlated endpoints. To understand the natural history of cancer, it would be informative to identify the prognostic factors of TTP and OS, as well as the association between TTP and OS through a single joint model. Once a joint model on the pair (OS, TTP) is established, TTP and other prognostic factors can be used to predict OS (Chap. 5).[2] For a methodological perspective, the pair (OS, TTP) can naturally explain the semi-competing risks relationship between two endpoints (Chap. 3).

The book also discusses a feature selection method for incorporating high-dimensional covariates, such as gene expressions, to the joint frailty-copula model. The book even aims to contribute to the development of personalized medicine by providing a dynamic survival prediction formula for a cancer patient, where copulas can effectively formulate the influence of tumour progression on survival.

To allow readers to apply the statistical methods of this book to their own data, we include case studies to demonstrate the R package *joint.Cox* (freely available from CRAN; https://cran.r-project.org/). With this package, readers can easily reproduce the results of our case studies, and they can analyze their data.

Our emphasis is placed on survival data arising from cancer research. Such data typically include survival endpoints, clinical covariates, and gene expressions collected on cancer patients. Accordingly, we provide case studies using survival data for cancer patients. Of course, statistical methods presented in this book can be applied to many branches of medical research, such as research on AIDS, cardio-vascular disorders, and neurological disorders. We also have seen that the statistical methods are useful outside medicine, especially in the field of reliability.

Use as a Textbook

This book may be used as a textbook for a one-semester course aimed at master students or a short course aimed at (bio) statisticians. Instructors (readers) may begin with Chap. 2. Chapter 1 can be assigned for preview. After that, instructors (readers) may proceed gradually to teach (learn) advanced statistical methods in Chaps. 3–5. Chapters 2 and 3 contain exercises useful for homework/self-study.

Chapter 2 provides an introduction to multivariate survival analysis to review many of the basic terms used throughout the book. Our review on the term *endpoint* is unique, which is not available in other textbooks on survival analysis. This

---

[2]However, it is not suitable to predict OS using endpoints such as DFS and PFS that include OS in their definitions (Chap. 2). While technically possible to fit the joint frailty-copula model on other the pairs, such as (OS, PFS) and (PFS, TTP), we shall not discuss this approach in this book.

chapter also reviews frailty models and copula models, the core elements of multivariate survival models. Studying these models can help understand the subsequent materials.

Chapter 3 introduces *semi-competing risks data* collected from multiple studies (meta-analysis). This type of data is getting easier to be obtained through free open source software and public data repository. However, relevant statistical methods are less discussed in the standard textbooks on survival analysis, though there are a number of journal articles on this theme in the last decade. The aim of Chap. 3 is to provide the basis for fitting the joint frailty-copula model to analyze semi-competing risks data.

Chapter 4 contains a feature selection method for high-dimensional gene expressions and the *compound covariate* method to be applied to the joint frailty-copula model. We detail the idea of compound covariate that was advocated by John Wilder Tukey in 1993 and its application to the joint frailty-copula model.

Chapter 5 considers a dynamic prediction method of predicting survival for a cancer patient under the joint frailty-copula model. The prediction formulas incorporate the genetic and clinical covariates collected on the patient entry as well as the tumour progression history evolving after the entry.

Chapter 6 collects additional remarks on the previous chapters, and several open problems for future research. This might help find research topics for students and researchers.

Use as a Reference Book

This book is designed to allow readers to read each chapter independently. Each chapter defines all terminologies and symbols with minimal references to other chapters. Also, each chapter provides a case study that helps readers understand how to apply the statistical methods and how to interpret the results. Readers who wish to analyze gene expression data may read Chap. 4. Readers who wish to develop a clinical prediction model may read Chap. 5. If readers feel difficulty in reading Chaps. 4 and 5, we suggest reading Chaps. 2 and 3 to build up basic skills.

Taoyuan City, Taiwan   Takeshi Emura
Nagoya, Japan   Shigeyuki Matsui
Bordeaux Cedex, France   Virginie Rondeau

Acknowledgements

We thank the series editor, Dr. Toshimitsu Hamasaki, for his invitation to write this book and his valuable comments on this book. We also thank Ms. Sayaka Shinohara for providing excellent figures for Chaps. 1, 3, and 5, and Mr. Jia-Han Shih for his effort to check the solutions to exercises. The contents of our book have been presented in a number of places, including *CM Statistics* conferences (2015 in London; 2016 in Seville; 2017 in London) and *2nd Pacific Rim Cancer Biostatistics Workshop* (2017 in Kanazawa), the *South Taiwan Statistics Conference* (in 2015, 2016, and 2017), and seminars arranged by Virginie Rondeau (2014 in University of Bordeaux), Hayashi Kenichi (2016 in Keio University), and Ha Il-Do (2018 in Pukyong National University). We thank all the organizers of the conferences and seminars. We also thank all those who listened to our speeches and gave us valuable comments, including David Cox, Helene Jacqmin-Gadda, Isao Yokota, Masataka Taguri, Mengjiao Peng, Roel Braekers, Motomi (Tomi) Mori, and Xiang Liming.

Emura T. is financially supported by Ministry of Science and Technology, Taiwan (MOST 107-2118-M-008-003-MY3). Matsui S. is financially supported by a Grant-in-Aid for Scientific Research (16II06299) and CREST, JST (JPMJCR1412) and from the Ministry of Education, Culture, Sports, Science and Technology of Japan. Rondeau V. is financially supported by the Fondation ARC pour la recherche sur le cancer, France.

Contents

Abbreviations

AIC	Akaike Information Criterion
CC	Compound Covariate
CI	Confidence Interval
DFS	Disease-Free Survival
FGM copula	Farlie-Gumbel-Morgenstern copula
GEO	Gene Expression Omnibus
IPD	Individual Patient Data
LCV	Likelihood Cross-Validation
OS	Overall Survival
PFS	Progression-Free Survival
RR	Relative Risk
SD	Standard Deviation
SE	Standard Error
TCGA	The Cancer Genome Atlas
TTP	Time-to-Tumour Progression

Notations

$a \in A$	An element a belonging to a set A
$\mathbf{a}'$	The transpose of a column vector $\mathbf{a}$
$E[X \mid Y]$	The conditional expectation of X given Y
$f : A \mapsto B$	A function from the domain A to the range B
$\dot{f}(x) = \mathrm{d}f(x)/\mathrm{d}x$	The first derivative of a function f
$\ddot{f}(x) = \mathrm{d}^2 f(x)/\mathrm{d}x^2$	The second derivative of a function f
$\arg\max_{\varphi} \ell(\varphi)$	The argument that maximizes a function ℓ
$N(0, \ 1)$	The standard normal distribution
$\mathbf{I}(\cdot)$	The indicator function: $\mathbf{I}(A) = 1$ if A is true, or $\mathbf{I}(A) = 0$ if A is false
$\Pr(A \mid B)$	The conditional probability of A given B
$\mathrm{tr}(\Omega)$	The trace of a square matrix Ω

Chapter 1
Setting the Scene

Abstract This chapter introduces the main theme of the book: statistical analysis of correlated endpoints using a joint/bivariate survival model. We first review statistical issues in the analysis of survival data involving correlated endpoints and censoring. We then illustrate our motivations of investigating the interrelationship between endpoints using joint/bivariate survival models. We finally illustrate how copulas and bivariate survival models have been grown through the literature.

Keywords Censoring · Competing risk · Cox regression · Dependent censoring · Endpoint · Informative dropout · Multivariate survival analysis · Overall survival · Time-to-tumour progression

1.1 Endpoints and Censoring

Survival analysis is a branch of statistics concerned with event times. In many examples of survival analysis, event times may be time-to-death as the name *survival* suggests. Time-to-death from any cause is termed *overall survival* (OS) which is considered as the most objective measure of patient health in cancer research (Chap. 2). More generally, event times can be *time-to-tumour progression* (TTP), *progression-free survival* (PFS), *disease-free survival* (DFS), and so on, which are all important measures of health status for cancer patients.

Multivariate survival analysis is a branch of survival analysis, which deals with two or more events per subject. For instance, one may observe both TTP and OS for a cancer patient. In analysis of such multivariate survival data, the key element is an appropriate account for dependence between event times. Throughout this book, we focus on *frailty* and *copulas* as main tools to model dependence between event times and to develop estimation and prediction methods.

Nowadays, statisticians and medical researchers can easily obtain multivariate survival data for patients through free open source software (e.g., R Bioconductor software) and public data repository (e.g., GEO and TCGA repositories). Many databases offer individual patient data containing two or more endpoints (OS, TTP, PFS, etc.) and a number of covariates (gene expressions, age, cancer stage, etc.).

© The Author(s), under exclusive license to Springer Nature Singapore Pte Ltd. 2019   1
T. Emura et al., *Survival Analysis with Correlated Endpoints*,
JSS Research Series in Statistics, https://doi.org/10.1007/978-981-13-3516-7_1

However, analyzing such multivariate survival data remains a challenging task as it requires model specifications on the association between endpoints. For instance, there exists a positive association between OS and TTP for cancer patients (Burzykowski et al 2008; Piedbois and Croswell 2008; Rondeau et al. 2015; Emura et al. 2017, 2018). To build a prognostic model for OS, multivariate survival models are required to stipulate the form of the joint distribution of OS and TTP. In addition, adequate statistical methods are required to estimate the degrees of association between OS and TTP.

Analysis of survival data is further complicated by *censoring*. If patient follow-up is terminated before observing endpoints, they are said to be *censored*. Censoring is unavoidable in survival data; the study has a planned end of follow-up, or patients may decide to withdraw from the study. If censoring mechanisms involve the dropout due to a worsening of the symptoms, it may introduce bias into statistical inference. Generally, if an endpoint of interest is censored by any mechanism related to the endpoint, this phenomenon shall be referred to *dependent censoring* (Emura and Chen 2018). If the endpoint of interest is TTP, one might regard death as a censoring event; however, statistical inference on TTP may be biased due to dependence between tumour progression and death. Most of the traditional survival analysis methods give a valid result under the *independent censoring assumption,* that is, censoring mechanisms are unrelated to the endpoint of interest.

The Cox proportional hazards regression model (Cox 1972) has been one of the traditional survival analysis tools among statisticians and medical researchers. The partial likelihood approach (Cox 1972) provides a statistical inference procedure for the Cox model. However, the Cox model with the partial likelihood approach is clearly insufficient to analyze multivariate survival data, such as the bivariate survival data in which TTP and OS are two endpoints of interest. In addition, it may *not* be a valid approach to fit the Cox model for TTP by treating death as independent censoring. This is because the independent censoring assumption made on the partial likelihood approach may be invalid. For a similar reason, it may not be a valid approach to fit the Cox model for OS if the censoring involves the dropout due to a worsening of the symptoms. Furthermore, if one wishes to study the link between TTP and OS, the Cox model for OS adjusted for TTP as a time-dependent covariate is not appropriate since the Cox model can only handle exogenous or external time-dependent covariates (that is, the covariate process develops independently of the event process). This is why the alternative framework of the joint/multivariate models for two time-to-event endpoints has been developed (Rondeau et al. 2015).

The book hopes to provide statistical methods that appropriately account for the issues that have just been mentioned.

1.2   Motivations for Investigating Correlated Endpoints

Researchers may demand a joint/bivariate survival model to specify the interrelationship between endpoints. This book introduces *frailty* and *copulas* as main tools for constructing a joint model. Listed below are specific motivations for adopting a joint model to deal with correlated endpoints.

1.2.1   Understanding Disease Progression Mechanisms

In clinical trials, researchers often evaluate the treatment effect on selected endpoints such as OS and TTP. Clearly, these endpoints are associated and evaluation of how TTP relates OS is important to understand disease progression mechanisms and to develop anti-cancer drugs (Sherrill et al. 2008; Michiels et al. 2009; Rondeau et al. 2015). In the medical literature, the treatment effect on endpoints is estimated by fitting the Cox model separately for each endpoint, but the results do not allow one to study the dependence among endpoints. With a joint/multivariate model that accounts for dependence among endpoints, the results give more insight into the natural history of the disease and may provide physicians with a useful patient management strategy dealing with multiple event risks. Chapter 3 introduces our recently developed approaches through the *joint frailty-copula model* between TTP and OS (Emura et al. 2017). Chapter 4 extends the joint frailty-copula model to incorporate high-dimensional covariates based on Tukey's compound covariate method (Matsui 2006; Emura et al. 2012, 2019). Building such a prognostic model with high-dimensional covariates is an urgent issue to promote personalized or predictive medicine through statistical methodologies (Matsui et al. 2015). Chapter 5 proposes a personalized prediction formula to predict OS according to TTP and covariates.

1.2.2   Dynamic Prediction of Death

In cancer studies, predicting risk of death is fundamental for improving patient care and treatment strategies. There is a great interest in *dynamic prediction* that predicts risk of death at a certain moment by utilizing the record of intermediate events (van Houwelingen and Putter 2011; Mauguen et al. 2013, 2015; Rondeau et al. 2017; Sène et al. 2016; Emura et al. 2018). For instance, dynamic prediction can utilize tumour progression histories (e.g., relapse) evolving over time to predict survival for an individual patient. Clearly, tumour progression histories are related to survival as a patient often encounters death immediately after tumour progression. This implies that the probability of death can substantially increases after experiencing tumour progression (Fig. 1.1). Accordingly, a bivariate survival model (joint model) for correlated endpoints is essential to build a prediction model. Such joint models for

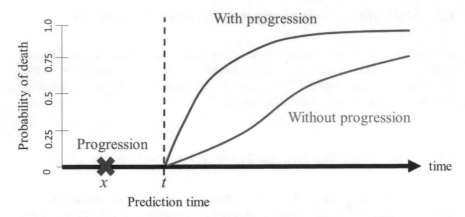

Fig. 1.1 The predicted probability of death can substantially increase after experiencing tumour progression. Prediction is made at time t according to tumour progression histories. If a patient experiences tumour progression before time t, TTP information x can be used for prediction. The details shall be discussed in Chap. 5

dependent endpoints have been developed under frailty models (Mauguen et al. 2013, 2015) and are utilized for the development of personalized medicine (Sène et al. 2016). Chapter 5 introduces a different approach based on the joint frailty-copula model, which allows one to utilize meta-analytic data.

1.2.3 Validating Surrogate Endpoints

Measuring dependence between endpoints is an essential process to validate surrogate endpoints to be adopted in clinical trials. The formal statistical validation is possible by using meta-analysis (Burzykowski et al. 2005; Shi and Sargent 2009; Rotolo et al. 2018). In meta-analytic studies, the process of validating surrogate endpoints utilizes two different kinds of dependency; study-level dependence and individual-level dependence (Buyse et al. 2008; Burzykowski et al. 2001, 2005).

A strong individual-level dependency between progression-free survival (PFS) and OS was found in patients with colorectal cancer (Buyse et al. 2008), head and neck cancer (Michiels et al. 2009), gastric cancer (Oba et al. 2013) and other cancers. A strong individual-level dependence between time-to-recurrence and OS was observed in advanced and early colon cancers (Alonso and Molenberghs 2008). These analyses adopted copulas to measure dependence between two endpoints. We shall discuss the topic of surrogate endpoints shortly as an important direction for future research in Chap. 6.

1.3   Copulas and Bivariate Survival Models: A Brief History

A *copula* is a function to link two random variables together to form a joint distribution. The concept of copulas was introduced by a mathematician, Abe Sklar, in his study of probabilistic metric space (Sklar 1959). From a modeling point of view, copulas allow one to create a dependence structure between two variables by specifying a copula function. Remarkably, a copula function does not restrict the structure of the marginal distributions. Consequently, measures of dependence, such as Kendall's tau, can be derived from a copula without influenced by the marginal distributions. More about copulas can be found in the book of Nelsen (2006).

Apparently, the applications of copulas in multivariate survival analysis became active after David George Clayton introduced his bivariate survival model (Clayton 1978). His work yielded one of the most important copulas for bivariate survival analysis, later known as *the Clayton copula*. The Clayton copula is a special case of *Archimedean copulas* (Genest and MacKay 1986) that contain several useful copulas, such as the Gumbel and Frank copulas. On the other hand, Clayton's model is also regarded as the gamma frailty model (Oakes 1989). More details shall be discussed in Chap. 2.

One of the most successful papers on copula-based survival models is Burzykowski et al. (2001) who developed the *two-step method* for analyzing dependence between two correlated endpoints. In the design of cancer clinical trials with surrogate endpoints, the current consensus is to base the copula-based validation approach using the two-step method (Burzykowski et al. 2005). An R package for implementing the two-step method is recently developed by Rotolo et al. (2018).

While the two-step approach considers dependence between two event times via copulas, their estimation algorithm relies on the assumption of independent censorship. An inconvenience occurs if one event censors the other. For instance, early death censors the occurrence of tumour progression, and hence, TTP is dependently censored by death. Hence, it is not a valid way to apply the two-step method by treating TTP and OS as bivariate event times subject to independent censoring. This problem is known as *competing risks* or *dependent censoring*. If one fits the Cox model to TTP endpoint by treating death as an independent censoring, the estimates of the effects of prognostic factors are systematically biased (Emura and Chen 2016, 2018; Moradian et al. 2017).

Fine et al. (2001) introduced the concept of *semi-competing risks* in which a terminal event censors a nonterminal event, but not vice versa. The statistical approach developed by Fine et al. (2001) provides a valid way to fit Clayton's model to data with TTP and OS. Their statistical approach was developed under Clayton's model and it was later extended to Archimedean copula models by Wang (2003). Chen (2012) further extended the copula models to implement semiparametric regression analysis on the transformation Cox model.

For a methodological point of view, copulas offer a unified strategy for modeling/analyzing survival data. For instance, the goodness-of-fit test of Emura et al. (2010) for Archimedean copulas is more general than that of Shih (1998) that is tailored for Clayton's model. The likelihood-based method of Chen (2012) for copulas is more general than the moment-based method of Fine et al. (2001) for Clayton's model.

Indeed, copula-based methods are adaptive to survival data with complex dependence structures, such as clustered survival data (Rotolo et al. 2013; Emura et al. 2017; Peng et al. 2018), dependent competing risks data (Lo and Wilke 2010; Chen 2010; de Uña-Álvarez and Veraverbeke 2013, 2017; Emura and Michimae 2017; Shih and Emura 2018), dependently censored data with one covariate (Braekers and Veraverbeke 2005) or high-dimensional covariates (Emura and Chen 2016), dependently truncated data (Chaieb et al. 2006; Emura and Murotani 2015; Emura and Pan 2017), multivariate survival data with complex association pattern (Barthel et al. 2018), and recurrent event data (Ling et al. 2016; Li et al. 2019).

In summary, copulas have provided flexible survival models and unified statistical methods. Here, copulas stipulate a dependence structure between two endpoints while they impose no restriction on their marginal distributions. Consequently, copulas provide measures of dependence, such as Kendall's tau, that are free from the model specifications of the marginal survival distributions. One can choose any copula that he/she likes from a large pool of existing copulas. One can also choose any specific type of regression models for marginal survival distribution, e.g., the Cox model with parametric or nonparametric baseline hazard function. This modeling strategy, which is adopted in this book, provides considerable flexibility/adaptability to different types of survival data. Copulas would continue to be the heart of modeling survival data with correlated endpoints.

References

Alonso A, Molenberghs G (2008) Evaluating time to cancer recurrence as a surrogate marker for survival from an information theory perspective. Stat Methods Med Res 17(5):497–504

Barthel N, Geerdens C, Killiches M, Janssen P, Czado C (2018) Vine copula based likelihood estimation of dependence patterns in multivariate event time data. Compt Stat Data Anal 117:109–127

Braekers R, Veraverbeke N (2005) A copula-graphic estimator for the conditional survival function under dependent censoring. Can J Stat 33:429–447

Burzykowski T, Buyse M, Piccart-Gebhart MJ et al (2008) Evaluation of tumor response, disease control, progression-free survival, and time to progression as potential surrogate end points in metastatic breast cancer. J Clin Oncol 26(12):1987–1992

Burzykowski T, Molenberghs G, Buyse M (eds) (2005) The Evaluation of Surrogate Endpoints. Springer, New York

Burzykowski T, Molenberghs G, Buyse M, Geys H, Renard D (2001) Validation of surrogate end points in multiple randomized clinical trials with failure time end points. Appl Stat 50(4):405–422

Buyse M, Burzykowski T, Michiels S, Carroll K (2008) Individual-and trial-level surrogacy in colorectal cancer. Stat Methods Med Res 17:467–475

Chaieb LL, Rivest LP, Abdous B (2006) Estimating survival under a dependent truncation. Biometrika 93(3):655–69

Chen YH (2010) Semiparametric marginal regression analysis for dependent competing risks under an assumed copula. J R Stat Soc Series B Stat Methodol 72:235–251

Chen YH (2012) Maximum likelihood analysis of semicompeting risks data with semiparametric regression models. Lifetime Data Anal 18:36–57

Clayton DG (1978) A model for association in bivariate life tables and its application in epidemiological studies of familial tendency in chronic disease incidence. Biometrika 65(1):141–151

Cox DR (1972) Regression models and life-tables (with discussion). J R Stat Soc Series B Stat Methodol 34:187–220

de Uña-Álvarez J, Veraverbeke N (2013) Generalized copula-graphic estimator. TEST 22(2):343–360

de Uña-Álvarez J, Veraverbeke N (2017) Copula-graphic estimation with left-truncated and right-censored data. Statistics 51(2):387–403

Emura T, Chen YH (2016) Gene selection for survival data under dependent censoring, a copula-based approach. Stat Methods Med Res 25(6):2840–2857

Emura T, Chen YH (2018) Analysis of survival data with dependent censoring, copula-based approaches, JSS Research Series in Statistics, Springer

Emura T, Chen YH, Chen HY (2012) Survival prediction based on compound covariate under Cox proportional hazard models. PLoS ONE 7(10):e47627. https://doi.org/10.1371/journal.pone.0047627

Emura T, Lin CW, Wang W (2010) A goodness-of-fit test for Archimedean copula models in the presence of right censoring. Compt Stat Data Anal 54:3033–3043

Emura T, Matsui S, Chen HY (2019) compound.Cox: univariate feature selection and compound covariate for predicting survival. Comput Methods Programs Biomed 168:21–37

Emura T, Michimae H (2017) A copula-based inference to piecewise exponential models under dependent censoring, with application to time to metamorphosis of salamander larvae. Environ Ecol Stat 24(1):151–173

Emura T, Murotani K (2015) An algorithm for estimating survival under a copula-based dependent truncation model. TEST 24(4):734–751

Emura T, Nakatochi M, Murotani K, Rondeau V (2017) A joint frailty-copula model between tumour progression and death for meta-analysis. Stat Methods Med Res 26(6):2649–2666

Emura T, Nakatochi M, Matsui S, Michimae H, Rondeau V (2018) Personalized dynamic prediction of death according to tumour progression and high-dimensional genetic factors: meta-analysis with a joint model. Stat Methods Med Res 27(9):2842–2858

Emura T, Pan CH (2017) Parametric likelihood inference and goodness-of-fit for dependently left-truncated data, a copula-based approach. Stat Pap. https://doi.org/10.1007/s00362-017-0947-z

Fine JP, Jiang H, Chappell R (2001) On semi-competing risks data. Biometrika 88:907–920

Genest C, MacKay J (1986) The joy of copulas: bivariate distributions with uniform marginals. The Am Stat 40(4):280–283

Lo SM, Wilke RA (2010) A copula model for dependent competing risks. J Roy Stat Soc Ser C (Appl Stat) 59(2):359–376

Li Z, Chinchilli VM, Wang M (2019) A Bayesian joint model of recurrent events and a terminal event. Biometrical Journal 61(1):187–202

Ling M, Tao Hu, Sun J (2016) Cox regression analysis of dependent interval-censored failure time data. Comput Stat Data Anal 103:79–90

Matsui S (2006) Predicting survival outcomes using subsets of significant genes in prognostic marker studies with microarrays. BMC Bioinformatics 7:156

Matsui S, Buyse M, Simon R (eds) (2015) Design and analysis of clinical trials for predictive medicine, vol 72. CRC Press, New York

Mauguen A, Rachet B, Mathoulin-Pélissier S et al (2013) Dynamic prediction of risk of death using history of cancer recurrences in joint frailty models. Stat Med 32(30):5366–5380

Mauguen A, Rachet B, Mathoulin-Pélissier S et al (2015) Validation of death prediction after breast cancer relapses using joint models. BMC Med Res Methodol 15(1):27

Michiels S, Le Maître A, Buyse M et al (2009) Surrogate endpoints for overall survival in locally advanced head and neck cancer: meta-analyses of individual patient data. Lancet Oncol 10(4):341–350

Moradian H, Denis Larocque D, Bellavance F (2017) Survival forests for data with dependent censoring. Stat Methods Med Res. https://doi.org/10.1177/0962280217727314

Nelsen RB (2006) An Introduction to Copulas, 2nd edn. Springer, New York

Oakes D (1989) Bivariate survival models induced by frailties. J Am Stat Assoc 84:487–493

Oba K, Paoletti X, Alberts S et al (2013) Disease-free survival as a surrogate for overall survival in adjuvant trials of gastric cancer: a meta-analysis. J Natl Cancer Inst 105(21):1600–1607

Peng M, Xiang L, Wang S (2018) Semiparametric regression analysis of clustered survival data with semicompeting risks. Compt Stat Data Anal 124:53–70

Piedbois P, Croswell MJ (2008) Surrogate endpoints for overall survival in advanced colorectal cancer: a clinician's perspective. Stat Methods Med Res 17(5):519–527

Rondeau V, Mauguen A, Laurent A, Berr C, Helmer C (2017) Dynamic prediction models for clustered and interval-censored outcomes: investigating the intra-couple correlation in the risk of dementia. Stat Methods Med Res 26(5):2168–2183

Rondeau V, Pignon JP, Michiels S (2015) A joint model for dependence between clustered times to tumour progression and deaths: a meta-analysis of chemotherapy in head and neck cancer. Stat Methods Med Res 24(6):711–729

Rotolo F, Legrand C, Van Keilegom I (2013) A simulation procedure based on copulas to generate clustered multi-state survival data. Comput Methods Programs Biomed 109(3):305–312

Rotolo F, Paoletti X. Michiels S (2018) surrosurv: an r package for the evaluation of failure time surrogate endpoints in individual patient data meta-analyses of randomized clinical trials. Comput Methods Programs Biomed 155:189–198

Sène M, Taylor JM, Dignam JJ et al (2016) Individualized dynamic prediction of prostate cancer recurrence with and without the initiation of a second treatment: development and validation. Stat Methods Med Res 25(6):2972–2991

Sherrill B, Amonker M, Wu Y et al (2008) Relationship between effects on time-to-disease progression and overall survival in studies of metastatic breast cancer. Br J Cancer 99:1542–1548

Shi Q, Sargent DJ (2009) Meta-analysis for the evaluation of surrogate endpoints in cancer clinical trials. Int J Clin Oncol 14(2):102–111

Shih JH (1998) A goodness-of-fit test for association in a bivariate survival model. Biometrika 85(1):189–200

Shih JH, Emura T (2018) Likelihood-based inference for bivariate latent failure time models with competing risks under the generalized FGM copula. Comput Stat 33(3):1293–1323

Sklar A (1959) Fonctions de répartition àn dimensions et leurs marges. Publications de l'Institut de Statistique de L'Université de Paris 8:229–231

van Houwelingen HC, Putter H (2011) Dynamic Prediction in Clinical Survival Analysis. CRC Press, New York

Wang W (2003) Estimating the association parameter for copula models under dependent censoring. J R Stat Soc Series B Stat Methodol 65(1):257–273

Chapter 2
Introduction to Multivariate Survival Analysis

Abstract This chapter introduces a framework for multivariate survival analysis that is used in later chapters. We first explain the concepts of endpoint and censoring in medical follow-up studies. Next, we review the basic tools in survival analysis, such as the survival/hazard function, Cox regression, and likelihood-based method. Finally, we introduce two major procedures for describing dependence among event times: (i) the shared frailty models for clustered survival data (ii) the copula models for bivariate survival data. We provide some exercises at the end of this chapter.

Keywords Censoring · Copula · Cox regression · Endpoint · Frailty · Independent censoring · Overall survival · Time-to-tumour progression

2.1 Endpoints and Censoring

In survival analysis, the term *survival time* refers to the time elapsed from an origin to the occurrence of an event. In many medical studies, the origin may be the time at study entry that can be the start of a medical treatment, the initiation of a randomized experiment, or the operation date of surgery. In epidemiological studies, the origin is often the date of birth. The event may be the occurrence of death, cancer relapse, or tumour progression, which depends on the research design.

The term *endpoint* has the same definition as survival time, but is more specifically used as a primary measure of evaluating medical treatments. Time-to-death is also called *overall survival*. For instance, if one is interested in measuring the effect of chemotherapy or radiotherapy in locally advanced head and neck cancer, the primary endpoint is overall survival (Michiels et al. 2009; Le Tourneau et al. 2009).

Several different endpoints have been employed to measure a clinically convincing effect of treatments or drugs for cancer patients (Pazdur 2008; Piedbois and Croswell 2008; Le Tourneau et al. 2009; Soria et al. 2010; Hamasaki et al. 2016). Endpoints should be well-defined and unambiguous measures that objectively assess clinically important aspects of a patient. The most popular endpoint is overall survival, which is precisely defined as follows:

© The Author(s), under exclusive license to Springer Nature Singapore Pte Ltd. 2019
T. Emura et al., *Survival Analysis with Correlated Endpoints*,
JSS Research Series in Statistics, https://doi.org/10.1007/978-981-13-3516-7_2

9

Definition 1 Overall survival (OS) is defined as the time elapsed from study entry to death from any cause.

Owing to the unambiguity of the definition of death, OS has been the gold standard endpoint in many cancer studies (Pazdur 2008; Shi and Sargent 2009; Michiels et al. 2009; Oba et al. 2013).

Another endpoint of interest is the elapsed time from study entry to any increase in tumour size, appearance of new tumour, or distant metastasis (collectively called *progression*):

Definition 2 Time-to-tumour progression (TTP) is defined as the time elapsed from study entry to the first evidence of tumour progression.

In cancer research, TTP may stand for time-to-progression rather than time-to-tumour progression. However, the distinction between time-to-progression and time-to-tumour progression is not always clear in the literature, and hence they may be used interchangeably. In either case, a careful and precise definition of "progression event" is necessary by following some guideline (e.g., RECIST guideline; Eisenhauer et al. 2009).

The occurrence of death is not considered as a tumour progression event. Hence, OS and TTP are distinct event times. The first occurring event between TTP and OS is referred to *progression-free survival* (PFS), i.e., PFS = min{OS, TTP}. Hence, OS and PFS are not distinct event times as OS is part of PFS. Since TTP may be shorter than OS in patients with cancer-related deaths, TTP and PFS generally allow faster clinical trials, compared with those evaluating OS.

Disease-free survival (DFS) is another endpoint defined as the time from a medical treatment until recurrence of disease or death from any cause. DFS is similar to PFS, but is more specifically used for the adjuvant setting after surgery or radiotherapy, where long survivors are expected.

The endpoints such as OS, TTP, PFS, and DFS are popular in applications of survival analysis to cancer research. The adequate choice of the endpoints depends on the type of diseases (or types of cancers), sample sizes (or powers), study period, and the goal of the research. Some discussions about OS, TTP, PFS, and DFS can be found in the medical literature (Pazdur 2008; Green et al. 2008; Soria et al. 2010; Cheema and Burkes 2013) and in the biostatistical literature (Rondeau et al. 2015; Emura et al. 2017, 2018; Matsui et al. 2015; Hamasaki et al. 2016; Sugimoto et al. 2017).

Unlike OS, the definitions of TTP, PFS, and DFS vary with the clinicians—i.e., the tumour progression may be defined by their own timing and assessment criteria. This often brings some ambiguity as a primary measure of evaluating a medical treatment. Hence, the definition of tumour progression or disease recurrence should clearly be described in the study protocol. In addition, tumour progression assessments generally should be verified by central reviewers blinded to the treatments under study, especially when the study is not blinded (e.g., in the absence of a placebo control).

In medical follow-up studies, OS for a patient is possibly censored by some mechanisms to terminate the studies. For example, a clinical trial typically has a predetermined follow-up period. Clinicians may not obtain OS information for those patients who are still alive after the study end. For another example, clinicians may fail to obtain OS if a patient drops out of (or withdraws from) the trial before he/she dies. In such circumstances, clinicians acquire partial information about OS as the elapsed time until the censoring point.

Definition 3 If OS is the primary endpoint, censoring time is defined as the time elapsed from study entry to the censoring event due to dropout (or withdrawal) from a study, or the end of a predetermined follow-up period. If TTP is the primary endpoint, the censoring event also includes death.

In the presence of censoring, clinicians can access either OS or censoring time, whichever comes first for a patient. OS is available if the patient dies during the follow-up. Alternatively, censoring time is available if the patient is alive at the end of the study period or at the time of dropout.

Similarly, PFS and DFS are subject to censoring due to the termination of follow-up or patients' early withdrawals. Unlike PFS and DFS, TTP can also be censored by death because TTP and OS are distinct event times as noted previously. Therefore, the use of TTP endpoint for cancer patients would be more effective than PFS and DFS in situations where the majority of deaths are unrelated to cancer.

Multivariate survival analysis is a branch of survival analysis that deals with more than one event times per subject. For instance, one may observe both TTP and OS for a cancer patient. In analysis of such multivariate survival data, the key element is an appropriate account for dependence between event times.

2.2 Basic Terminologies

This section summarizes basic terminologies and notations used in survival analysis.
Consider *random variables*, defined as

- X: event time
- C: censoring time

Due to *censoring*, either one of X or C is observed. One can observe X if an event comes faster than censoring ($X \leq C$). On the other hand, one cannot exactly observe X if censoring comes faster than an event ($X > C$). Even if the exact value of X is unknown for the censored case, X is known to be greater than C. What we observe are the first occurring time ($\min\{X, C\}$) and the censoring status ($X \leq C$ or $X > C$).

Survival data consist of $\{(T_i, \delta_i); i = 1, \ldots, n\}$, where

- T_i: event time or censoring time whichever comes first,
- δ_i: censoring indicator ($\delta_i = 1$ if T_i is event time, or $\delta_i = 0$ if T_i is censoring time).

One can write $T_i = \min\{X_i, C_i\}$ and $\delta_i = \mathbf{I}(X_i \leq C_i)$, where $\mathbf{I}(\cdot)$ is the indicator function.

Survival data often include *covariates*, such as gender, tumour size, and cancer stage. In medical applications, covariates are usually *prognostic factors* that are associated with event time. With covariates, the dataset consists of $\{(T_i, \delta_i, \mathbf{Z}_i); i = 1, \ldots, n\}$, where

- $\mathbf{Z}_i = (Z_{i1}, \ldots, Z_{ip})'$: p-dimensional covariates.

Throughout this chapter, we impose the following assumption:

Independent censoring assumption*: X and C are conditionally independent given $\mathbf{Z}$.*

This assumption is imposed on most statistical methods for analyzing survival data, such as Cox regression (Sect. 2.3). If the independent censoring assumption does not hold, X can be *dependently censored by C*. However, throughout this book, the symbol C always represents censoring time that satisfies the independent censoring assumption.

The *survival function* is defined as $S(t|\mathbf{Z}_i) \equiv \Pr(X_i > t|\mathbf{Z}_i)$ that is the probability that the patient with covariates $\mathbf{Z}_i$ is event-free at time t. This is the *patient-level survival function* as it is conditionally on patient characteristics. The survival function at $\mathbf{Z}_i = \mathbf{0}$ is called the *baseline survival function* and denoted as $S_0(t) = S(t|\mathbf{Z}_i = \mathbf{0})$.

Hereafter, we suppose that $S(t|\mathbf{Z}_i)$ is continuous and differentiable in t. The instantaneous probability of experiencing an event between t and $t + dt$ is $S(t|\mathbf{Z}_i) - S(t + dt|\mathbf{Z}_i)$, where dt is an infinitely small number. Since this probability is equal to zero, we consider the *rate* by dividing by dt such that

$$f(t|\mathbf{Z}_i) = \frac{S(t|\mathbf{Z}_i) - S(t + dt|\mathbf{Z}_i)}{dt} = -\frac{dS(t|\mathbf{Z}_i)}{dt}.$$

This is the *density function*.

The density function represents the frequency of events at time t. While the density is an important measure in epidemiology or demography, it is not frequently used in prognostic analysis of a patient. This is because a patient or clinician is more interested in the *risk* than the frequency.

We formulate the risk of a patient as the instantaneous event rate between t and $t + dt$ given that the patient is surviving at time t. The risk, expressed as a function of t, is called the *hazard function*:

Definition 4 The hazard function is defined as

$$\lambda(t|\mathbf{Z}_i) \equiv \frac{\Pr(t \le X_i < t + dt | X_i \ge t, \mathbf{Z}_i)}{dt} = -\frac{d}{dt} \log S(t|\mathbf{Z}_i).$$

The cumulative hazard function is defined as

$$\Lambda(t|\mathbf{Z}_i) = \int_0^t \lambda(u|\mathbf{Z}_i) du.$$

The hazard function at $\mathbf{Z}_i = \mathbf{0}$ is called the *baseline hazard function* and denoted as $\lambda_0(t) = \lambda(t|\mathbf{Z}_i = \mathbf{0})$. Also, the baseline cumulative hazard function is defined as $\Lambda_0(t) = \int_0^t \lambda_0(u) du$.

The survival function and the cumulative hazard function is related through $S(t|\mathbf{Z}_i) = \exp\{-\Lambda(t|\mathbf{Z}_i)\}$. The hazard function is written as $\lambda(t|\mathbf{Z}_i) = f(t|\mathbf{Z}_i)/S(t|\mathbf{Z}_i)$.

A *parametric model* is defined by a survival function or hazard function that has a specified distributional form such as the exponential, Weibull, and log-normal distributions. In parametric models, the effects of covariates on survival also have a specific form. An example is an Weibull model $S(t|\mathbf{Z}_i) = \exp(-\lambda t^\nu e^{\boldsymbol{\beta}' \mathbf{Z}_i})$, $t \ge 0$, where $\lambda > 0$ is a scale parameter, $\nu > 0$ is a shape parameter, and $\boldsymbol{\beta}$ are regression coefficients. It can be shown that $S(t|\mathbf{Z}_i) = S_0(t)^{\exp(\boldsymbol{\beta}' \mathbf{Z}_i)}$ for $t \ge 0$, where $S_0(t) = S(t|\mathbf{Z}_i = \mathbf{0}) = \exp(-\lambda t^\nu)$ is the baseline survival function. With this model, the effects of the covariates on survival is captured by $\boldsymbol{\beta}$.

A *semi-parametric model* is defined by a survival function or hazard function that has a specified form of covariate effects on survival without a specified distributional form. Semi-parametric models are more flexible and usually fit better to data than parametric models.

To make statistical inference on semi-parametric models, some mild assumptions should still be made for the unspecified part. For instance, the baseline survival function $S_0(\cdot)$ is assumed to be a decreasing step function with jumps at observed times of death, or the baseline hazard function $\lambda_0(\cdot)$ is assumed to be a weighted sum of spline basis functions. In either case, these assumptions do not restrict too much the shape of the survival or hazard function by allowing a large number of parameters to be determined by data.

Unfortunately, parametric models, such as the exponential, Weibull and log-normal models, may not adequately fit survival data from cancer patients. This implies that survival experience of cancer patients do not show a simple pattern probably because they may experience complex treatment regimens and disease progression. This is why semi-parametric models are more useful and widely applied in medical research. One may still accept the assumptions that the hazard function is continuous, does not abruptly change over time, and smooth (continuously differentiable). Hazard models with cubic splines meet these assumptions without restricting too much the shape of the hazard function (see Sect. 2.4.1 for more details).

2.3 Cox Regression

The hazard function is a sensible measure for describing the risk of experiencing an event, and hence can be used for prognostic analysis for a patient. It is then natural to incorporate the effect of covariates into the hazard function.

> **Definition 5** The Cox proportional hazards model (Cox 1972) is defined as
>
> $$\lambda(t|\mathbf{Z}_i) = \lambda_0(t)\exp(\boldsymbol{\beta}'\mathbf{Z}_i),$$
>
> where $\boldsymbol{\beta} = (\beta_1, \ldots, \beta_p)'$ are unknown coefficients and $\lambda_0(\cdot)$ is an unknown baseline hazard function.

The Cox model states that all patients share the same time-trend function $\lambda_0(t)$. An important property of the Cox model is that the form of $\lambda_0(\cdot)$ is unspecified, meaning that the model is semi-parametric. Hence, the Cox model offers greater flexibility over parametric models that specify the form of $\lambda_0(\cdot)$. The Cox model is also specified as $S(t|\mathbf{Z}_i) = S_0(t)^{\exp(\boldsymbol{\beta}'\mathbf{Z}_i)}$ for $t \geq 0$, where the form of $S_0(t)$ is unspecified.

Let Z_i be a dichotomous covariate, such as gender with $Z_i = 1$ for male and $Z_i = 0$ for female. Under the Cox model $\lambda(t|Z_i) = \lambda_0(t)\exp(\beta Z_i)$, the *relative risk* (RR) is defined as

$$\text{RR} = \frac{\lambda(t|Z_i = 1)}{\lambda(t|Z_i = 0)} = \exp(\beta).$$

For instance, the value $\text{RR} = 2$ implies that the event rate under $Z_i = 1$ is twice the event rate under $Z_i = 0$.

Let Z_i be a continuous covariate, such as a gene expression. Under the Cox model $\lambda(t|Z_i) = \lambda_0(t)\exp(\beta Z_i)$, if the scale of Z_i is standardized (to be mean $= 0$ and SD $= 1$), the value $\exp(\beta)$ is interpreted as the RR for a one SD increase in Z_i. That is,

$$\text{RR} = \frac{\lambda(t|Z_i + 1)}{\lambda(t|Z_i)} = \exp(\beta).$$

Under the Cox model, one can use survival data $\{(T_i, \delta_i, \mathbf{Z}_i); i = 1, \ldots, n\}$ to estimate $\boldsymbol{\beta}$. Let $R_i = \{\ell : T_\ell \geq T_i\}$ be the *risk set* that contains patients *at-risk* at time T_i. The *partial likelihood estimator* $\hat{\boldsymbol{\beta}} = (\hat{\beta}_1, \ldots, \hat{\beta}_p)'$ is defined by maximizing the *partial likelihood function* (Cox 1972)

$$L(\boldsymbol{\beta}) = \prod_{i=1}^{n} \left(\frac{\exp(\boldsymbol{\beta}'\mathbf{Z}_i)}{\sum_{\ell \in R_i} \exp(\boldsymbol{\beta}'\mathbf{Z}_\ell)} \right)^{\delta_i}.$$

The estimator $\hat{\boldsymbol{\beta}}$ is consistent when the independent censoring assumption holds and the model specification is correct (Fleming and Harrington 1991). If the independent censoring assumption does not hold, $\hat{\boldsymbol{\beta}}$ is a biased estimate for the true regression coefficients (Emura and Chen 2016, 2018).

The log-partial likelihood is

$$\ell(\boldsymbol{\beta}) = \log L(\boldsymbol{\beta}) = \sum_{i=1}^{n} \delta_i \left[\boldsymbol{\beta}'\mathbf{Z}_i - \log \left\{ \sum_{\ell \in R_i} \exp(\boldsymbol{\beta}'\mathbf{Z}_\ell) \right\} \right].$$

The derivatives of $\ell(\boldsymbol{\beta})$ give the *score function*,

$$\mathbf{S}(\boldsymbol{\beta}) = \frac{\partial \ell(\boldsymbol{\beta})}{\partial \boldsymbol{\beta}} = \sum_{i=1}^{n} \delta_i \left[\mathbf{Z}_i - \frac{\sum_{\ell \in R_i} \mathbf{Z}_\ell \exp(\boldsymbol{\beta}'\mathbf{Z}_\ell)}{\sum_{\ell \in R_i} \exp(\boldsymbol{\beta}'\mathbf{Z}_\ell)} \right].$$

The second-order derivatives of $\ell(\boldsymbol{\beta})$ constitute the *Hessian matrix*,

$$H(\boldsymbol{\beta}) = \frac{\partial^2 \ell(\boldsymbol{\beta})}{\partial \boldsymbol{\beta} \partial \boldsymbol{\beta}'}$$

$$= -\sum_{i=1}^{n} \delta_i \left[\frac{\sum_{\ell \in R_i} \mathbf{Z}_\ell \mathbf{Z}_\ell' \exp(\boldsymbol{\beta}'\mathbf{Z}_\ell)}{\sum_{\ell \in R_i} \exp(\boldsymbol{\beta}'\mathbf{Z}_\ell)} - \frac{\sum_{\ell \in R_i} \mathbf{Z}_\ell \exp(\boldsymbol{\beta}'\mathbf{Z}_\ell)}{\sum_{\ell \in R_i} \exp(\boldsymbol{\beta}'\mathbf{Z}_\ell)} \right.$$

$$\left. \left\{ \frac{\sum_{\ell \in R_i} \mathbf{Z}_\ell \exp(\boldsymbol{\beta}'\mathbf{Z}_\ell)}{\sum_{\ell \in R_i} \exp(\boldsymbol{\beta}'\mathbf{Z}_\ell)} \right\}' \right].$$

Interval estimates for $\boldsymbol{\beta}$ are obtained by applying the asymptotic theory (Fleming and Harrington 1991). The *information matrix* is defined as $i(\hat{\boldsymbol{\beta}}) = -H(\hat{\boldsymbol{\beta}})$. The standard error (SE) of $\hat{\beta}_j$ is $\mathrm{SE}(\hat{\beta}_j) = \sqrt{\{i^{-1}(\hat{\boldsymbol{\beta}})\}_{jj}}$, where $\{i^{-1}(\hat{\boldsymbol{\beta}})\}_{jj}$ is the j-th diagonal element of the inverse information matrix. The 95% confidence interval (CI) is $\hat{\beta}_j \pm 1.96 \times \mathrm{SE}(\hat{\beta}_j)$. The Wald test for the null hypothesis $H_0 : \beta_j = 0$ is based on the Z-value $z = \hat{\beta}_j / \mathrm{SE}(\hat{\beta}_j)$. The P-value is computed as $\Pr(|Z| > |z|)$, where $Z \sim N(0, 1)$.

2.3.1   R Survival Package

We shall briefly introduce the R package *survival* to perform Cox regression.

As a running example, we use a dataset consisting of $n = 58$ ovarian cancer patients obtained from "Study 2" that shall be mentioned in Sect. 2.5. The event time of interest is time-to-recurrence after surgery. In the data, 48 patients experience cancer recurrence and other 10 patients are censored. The covariate is a binary variable ($Z_j = 0$ vs. $Z_j = 1$) on the residual tumour size at surgery (≤ 1 cm vs. >1 cm).

After installing the package, we enter event time t_i, censoring indicator δ_i, and covariate Z_i for $n = 58$ patients. Then, we run the codes:

```
library(survival)
t.event=c(385, 2582, 175, 162, 860, 3025, 454, 89, 252, 30, 401, 505, 511, 494, 195,
          31, 242, 2195, 2282, 309, 3315, 387, 287, 367, 542, 165, 31, 2246, 481, 1003,
          380, 367, 342, 265, 480, 664, 4208, 321, 431, 929, 125, 328, 3644, 811, 872,
          804, 580, 298, 12, 282, 218, 114, 566, 803, 265, 407, 208, 309) ## event times
event=c(1, 1, 1, 1, 1, 1, 1, 1, 1, 1, 1, 1, 1, 1, 1, 0, 1, 1, 0, 0, 1, 0, 0, 1, 1, 1, 1, 1, 1, 0, 1, 1, 1,
        1, 1, 1, 1, 0, 1, 1, 1, 0, 1, 0, 1, 1, 1, 1, 1, 1, 1, 1, 1, 1, 1, 1, 0, 1) ## censoring indicators
Z=c(1, 0, 1, 0; 0, 0, 0, 0, 1, 0, 1, 1, 1, 1, 1, 1, 1, 0, 0, 1, 1, 0, 0, 0, 0, 1, 1, 0, 0, 0, 0,
     1, 1, 0, 1, 1, 0, 1, 0, 0, 1, 1, 0, 1, 1, 1, 1, 1, 1, 1, 1, 1, 1, 0, 0, 0, 1, 0, 1) ## covariates
coxph(Surv(t.event,event)~Z)
```

Below are the outputs:

```
> coxph(Surv(t.event,event)~Z)
Call:
coxph(formula = Surv(t.event, event) ~ Z)

     coef   exp(coef)  se(coef)   z      p
Z   0.849   2.338      0.307      2.76   0.0057

Likelihood ratio test=7.9  on 1 df, p=0.00495
n= 58, number of events= 48
```

The results on Cox regression show $\hat{\beta} = 0.849$, $\mathrm{RR} = \exp(\hat{\beta}) = 2.338$, $\mathrm{SE}(\hat{\beta}) = 0.307$, and $z = \hat{\beta}/\mathrm{SE}(\hat{\beta}) = 2.76$. The P-value of the Wald test is 0.0057, and hence the residual tumour size is significantly associated with time-to-recurrence. The result implies that patients having a residual tumour (>1 cm) are more than twice as likely to experience cancer relapse after surgery. Hence, the residual tumour would be an important prognostic factor for cancer recurrence.

2.4   Likelihood-Based Method

This section considers likelihood-based methods for analyzing the dataset $\{(T_i, \delta_i, \mathbf{Z}_i); i = 1, \ldots, n\}$. These methods are applicable to both parametric and semi-parametric models, and hence, provide more general tools than the partial like-lihood method.

Event time X_i and censoring time C_i are related to the observation $(T_i, \ \delta_i)$ through

- $X_i = T_i$ and $C_i > T_i$ if $\delta_i = 1$,
- $X_i > T_i$ and $C_i = T_i$ if $\delta_i = 0$.

Each patient experiences either one of the two cases. Hence, the probability of observing the data ($T_i, \ \delta_i, \ \mathbf{Z}_i$) for the i-th patient is

$$L_i = \Pr(X_i = T_i, C_i > T_i | \mathbf{Z}_i)^{\delta_i} \Pr(X_i > T_i, C_i = T_i | \mathbf{Z}_i)^{1-\delta_i}.$$

This is the likelihood of binary outcomes. Under the independent censoring assumption,

$$
\begin{aligned}
L_i &= [\Pr(X_i = T_i | \mathbf{Z}_i) \Pr(C_i > T_i | \mathbf{Z}_i)]^{\delta_i} [\Pr(C_i = T_i | \mathbf{Z}_i) \Pr(X_i > T_i | \mathbf{Z}_i)]^{1-\delta_i} \\
&= [f_X(T_i | \mathbf{Z}_i) S_C(T_i | \mathbf{Z}_i)]^{\delta_i} [f_C(T_i | \mathbf{Z}_i) S_X(T_i | \mathbf{Z}_i)]^{1-\delta_i} \\
&= [f_X(T_i | \mathbf{Z}_i)^{\delta_i} S_X(T_i | \mathbf{Z}_i)^{1-\delta_i}][f_C(T_i | \mathbf{Z}_i)^{1-\delta_i} S_C(T_i | \mathbf{Z}_i)^{\delta_i}].
\end{aligned}
$$

where $S_X(t | \mathbf{Z}_i) = \Pr(X_i > t | \mathbf{Z}_i)$, $f_X(t | \mathbf{Z}_i) = -dS_X(t | \mathbf{Z}_i)/dt$, $S_C(t | \mathbf{Z}_i) = \Pr(C_i > t | \mathbf{Z}_i)$, and $f_C(t | \mathbf{Z}_i) = -dS_C(t | \mathbf{Z}_i)/dt$. In addition to the independent censoring assumption, we further impose the following assumption:

> **Non-informative censoring assumption**: $S_C(t | \mathbf{Z}_i)$ does not contain any parameters related to $S_X(t | \mathbf{Z}_i)$.

Under the non-informative censoring assumption, the term $f_C(T_i | \mathbf{Z}_i)^{1-\delta_i} S_C(T_i | \mathbf{Z}_i)^{\delta_i}$ can be ignored. Therefore, the likelihood function is redefined as

$$L = \prod_{i=1}^{n} f_X(T_i | \mathbf{Z}_i)^{\delta_i} S_X(T_i | \mathbf{Z}_i)^{1-\delta_i} = \prod_{i=1}^{n} \lambda_X(T_i | \mathbf{Z}_i)^{\delta_i} \exp[-\Lambda_X(T_i | \mathbf{Z}_i)], \quad (2.1)$$

The log-likelihood is

$$\ell = \log L = \sum_{i=1}^{n} [\delta_i \log \lambda_X(T_i | \mathbf{Z}_i) - \Lambda_X(T_i | \mathbf{Z}_i)].$$

Independent censoring and non-informative censoring are mathematically different concepts. However, independent censoring in real-world applications usually implies non-informative censoring. An artificial or unusual example may exist for informative but independent censoring (p. 150 of Andersen et al. 1993; p. 196 of Kalbfleisch and Prentice 2002). Independent censoring is more crucial assumption than non-informative censoring since dependent censoring leads to bias in estimation (Emura and Chen 2018).

Suppose that the log-likelihood is written as $\ell(\varphi)$, where φ is a vector of parameters. Then, the maximum likelihood estimator (MLE) is defined by $\hat{\varphi} = \arg\max_{\varphi} \ell(\varphi)$. The first derivatives of the log-likelihood give the *score function*, $\mathbf{S}(\varphi) = \partial\ell(\varphi)/\partial\varphi$. The second derivatives of the log-likelihood give the Hessian matrix $H(\varphi) = \partial^2\ell(\varphi)/\partial\varphi\partial\varphi'$. The MLE $\hat{\varphi}$ is obtained from the Newton–Raphson algorithm

$$\varphi^{(k+1)} = \varphi^{(k)} - H^{-1}(\varphi^{(k)})\mathbf{S}(\varphi^{(k)}), \quad k = 0, 1, \ldots.$$

Interval estimates for φ follow from the asymptotic theory of MLEs. The *information matrix* is defined as $i(\hat{\varphi}) = -H(\hat{\varphi})$. For the j-th component $\hat{\phi}_j$ of $\hat{\varphi}$, the standard error (SE) is $\mathrm{SE}(\hat{\phi}_j) = \sqrt{\{i^{-1}(\hat{\varphi})\}_{jj}}$, where $\{i^{-1}(\hat{\varphi})\}_{jj}$ is the j-th diagonal element of the inverse information matrix. The 95% CI is $\hat{\phi}_j \pm 1.96 \times \mathrm{SE}(\hat{\phi}_j)$.

2.4.1 Spline and Penalized Likelihood

We consider a proportional hazards model $\lambda(t|\mathbf{Z}_i) = \lambda_0(t;\mathbf{h})\exp(\beta'\mathbf{Z}_i)$, where the baseline hazard function is parametrically specified by a vector $\mathbf{h}$. Letting $\varphi = (\mathbf{h}, \beta)$, the log-likelihood is written as

$$\ell(\varphi) = \sum_{i=1}^{n} [\delta_i\{\log\lambda_0(T_i;\mathbf{h}) + \beta'\mathbf{Z}_i\} - \Lambda_0(T_i;\mathbf{h})\exp(\beta'\mathbf{Z}_i)].$$

If the dimension of $\mathbf{h}$ is high, the baseline hazard function is a complex function of t and difficult to interpret. In this case, one may wish to constrain the complexity of the hazard function. A popular way to quantify the complexity of a function f is through the *roughness* defined as $\int \ddot{f}(t)^2 dt$, where $\ddot{f}(t) = \mathrm{d}^2 f(t)/\mathrm{d}t^2$. We then maximize the likelihood while minimizing the roughness through a *penalized likelihood*

$$\ell(\varphi) - \kappa \int \ddot{\lambda}_0(t;\mathbf{h})^2 dt.$$

where $\kappa > 0$ is a given value, called a *smoothing parameter*.

A penalized likelihood is particularly useful for the spline-based method. The spline method allows for a flexible hazard function that is difficult to be achieved by parametric models such as the Weibull model. The spline method is also known for its computational effectiveness because the spline basis functions are easy to differentiate and integrate (Ramsay 1988).

We specify the baseline hazard function as $\lambda_0(t;\mathbf{h}) = \sum_{\ell=1}^{L} h_\ell M_\ell(t)$, where h_ℓ's are positive parameters and $M_\ell(t)$'s are called the M-spline basis functions (Ramsay 1988). The number of bases L also represents the number of free parameters. One has the baseline cumulative hazard function $\Lambda_0(t; \mathbf{h}) = \sum_{\ell=1}^{L} h_\ell I_\ell(t)$ and the baseline survival function $S_0(t; \mathbf{h}) = \exp\left[-\sum_{\ell=1}^{L} h_\ell I_\ell(t)\right]$, where $I_l(t)$'s are integrations of $M_l(t)$'s, called the I-spline basis functions.

To compute the spline basis functions, one needs to specify the knots and the range of t. One of the simplest ways is to set the range $t \in [\xi_1, \xi_3]$ for the equally spaced knots $\xi_1 < \xi_2 < \xi_3$, where $\xi_1 = \min(T_j)$, $\xi_3 = \max(T_j)$, and $\xi_2 = (\xi_1 + \xi_3)/2$. Figure 2.1 displays the M- and I-spline basis functions with $L = 5$ and the knots $\xi_1 = 1, \xi_2 = 2$, and $\xi_3 = 3$. The *joint.Cox* package (Emura 2019) provides functions *M.spline()* for $M_\ell(t)$ and *I.spline()* for $I_\ell(t)$ for $L = 5$. The expressions of $M_\ell(t)$ and $I_\ell(t)$ are given in Appendix A.

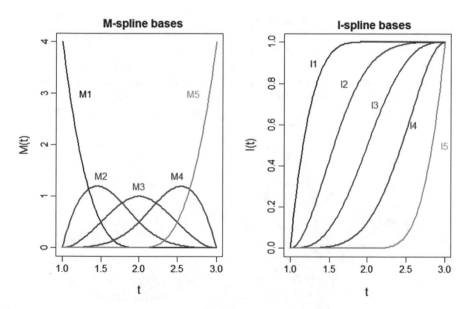

Fig. 2.1 M-spline basis functions (left-panel) and I-spline basis functions (right-panel) with knots $\xi_1 = 1, \xi_2 = 2$, and $\xi_3 = 3$

The *joint.Cox* R package (Emura 2019) provides a function *splineCox.reg()* to compute penalized MLEs. The function automatically selects the optimal value of κ among the user-specified grid points for κ. Since the choice of the grid points is not obvious, some graphical diagnostic tools are necessary, which shall be detailed in Chap. 3. Finally, the penalized likelihood estimator is defined as

$$(\hat{\boldsymbol{\beta}}^{\text{PL}}, \hat{\mathbf{h}}^{\text{PL}}) = \arg\max\left\{\ell(\boldsymbol{\beta}, \mathbf{h}) - \hat{\kappa} \int \ddot{\lambda}_0(t; \mathbf{h})^2 dt\right\},$$

where $\hat{\kappa}$ is the optimal value. Usually, the value of $\hat{\boldsymbol{\beta}}^{\text{PL}}$ is close to the partial likelihood estimator $\hat{\boldsymbol{\beta}}$.

2.5   Clustered Survival Data

Shared frailty models are useful to incorporate unexplained heterogeneity in the risks of experiencing an event for patients. For instance, we shall consider a multicenter analysis, where patients are collected from different hospitals. Obviously, some hospitals perform well while others perform poorly in terms of prolonging survival of their patients. In shared frailty models, it is assumed that each hospital has its own unobserved factor (called the frailty term) influencing the risks of all patients in the hospital. Hence, the patients in the same hospital *share* the same frailty term. Consequently, the study population may be regarded as a mixture of frail patients (in a hospital with a high frailty term) and robust patients (in a hospital with a low frailty term).

Individual patient data (IPD) meta-analysis is based on patients collected from different studies (Fig. 2.2). By replacing the term "center" to "study", IPD meta-analysis is essentially equivalent to multicenter analysis.

Figure 2.2 shows meta-analytic data collected from four different studies. The data provide time-to-recurrence for 912 surgically treated patients with ovarian cancer. One can observe the heterogeneity of relapse (recurrence) rates among the four studies, with highest being Study 2 (83%) and the lowest being Study 4 (49%).

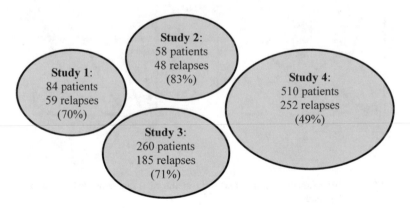

Fig. 2.2   Meta-analytic data combining four different studies of ovarian cancer patients (Ganzfried et al. 2013; Emura et al. 2018). The data is available in the *joint.Cox* R package (Emura 2019)

In both the IPD meta-analysis and multicenter analysis, it is customary to account for heterogeneity by means of random effects, called frailty. The gamma frailty distribution has been routinely applied to account for the heterogeneity, where the variance of the gamma distribution measures the degree of heterogeneity (Duchateau et al. 2002; Rondeau et al. 2015; Emura et al. 2017, 2018).

Instead of "study" or "center", we shall use a more general term "cluster" to represent the study unit. This allows one to think more general and broad applications encountered in medical studies, where a cluster is a well-defined collection of patients. In some family-based studies, a cluster may be a married couple (Rondeau et al. 2017), or a family containing more than one member (Rodríguez-Girondo et al. 2018).

2.5.1 Shared Frailty Model

We consider a dataset consisting of G independent clusters with the i-th cluster containing N_i patients. For $i = 1, 2, \ldots, G$ and $j = 1, 2, \ldots, N_i$, let X_{ij} be event time and $\mathbf{Z}_{ij}$ be a vector of covariates. For instance, the meta-analytic data of ovarian cancer patients contain $G = 4$ clusters, and each cluster has $N_1 = 84$, $N_2 = 58$, $N_3 = 260$, and $N_4 = 510$ patients (total 912 patients).

In the shared frailty models, the heterogeneity of the event rates is specified by multiplying a frailty term to the Cox model:

Definition 6 The shared frailty model is defined on the hazard function for the j-th patient in the i-th cluster:

$$\lambda_{ij}(t|u_i, \mathbf{Z}_{ij}) = u_i \lambda_0(t) \exp(\boldsymbol{\beta}'\mathbf{Z}_{ij}),$$

where $\boldsymbol{\beta} = (\beta_1, \ldots, \beta_p)'$ are unknown coefficients, $\lambda_0(\cdot)$ is an unknown baseline hazard function, and $u_i > 0$, $i = 1, 2, \ldots, G$, are unobserved frailty terms.

The most popular choice for the frailty distribution is the gamma density

$$f_\eta(u) = \frac{1}{\Gamma(1/\eta)\eta^{1/\eta}} u^{1/\eta - 1} \exp\left(-\frac{u}{\eta}\right), \quad \eta > 0, \ u > 0.$$

The mean and variance are $E_\eta(u_i) = 1$ and $\mathrm{Var}_\eta(u_i) = \eta$.

A high-risk cluster is expressed as $u_i > 1$, and a low-risk cluster is expressed as $0 < u_i < 1$. Hence, the variance parameter η represents the amount of heterogeneity in the risk of the event. The limit $\eta \to 0$ corresponds to the absence of heterogeneity. Note that the value of u_i is unobserved (i.e., u_i is a latent variable).

In the shared frailty models, it is assumed that X_{ij}, $j = 1, 2, \ldots, N_i$ are conditionally independent given u_i. Hence, the joint survival function given u_i is

$$\Pr(X_{ij} > x_{ij}, j = 1, 2, \ldots, N_i | u_i, \mathbf{Z}_{ij}, j = 1, 2, \ldots, N_i)$$

$$= \prod_{j=1}^{N_i} \Pr(X_{ij} > x_{ij}|u_i, \mathbf{Z}_{ij}) = \exp\left[-u_i \sum_{j=1}^{N_i} \Lambda_0(x_{ij}) \exp(\boldsymbol{\beta}'\mathbf{Z}_{ij})\right].$$

If we integrate out the unobserved u_i, we have the joint survival function

$$\Pr(X_{ij} > x_{ij}, j = 1, 2, \ldots, N_i | \mathbf{Z}_{ij}, j = 1, 2, \ldots, N_i)$$

$$= \int_0^\infty \exp\left[-u \sum_{j=1}^{N_i} \Lambda_0(x_{ij}) \exp(\boldsymbol{\beta}' \mathbf{Z}_{ij}) \right] f_\eta(u) du = \varphi_\eta\left[\sum_{j=1}^{N_i} \Lambda_0(x_{ij}) \exp(\boldsymbol{\beta}' \mathbf{Z}_{ij}) \right],$$

where $\varphi_\eta(s) = \int_0^\infty \exp(-su) f_\eta(u) du$ is the Laplace transform of $f_\eta(\cdot)$. Similarly, the marginal survival function is $\Pr(X_{ij} > x_{ij} | \mathbf{Z}_{ij}) = \varphi_\eta[\Lambda_0(x_{ij}) \exp(\boldsymbol{\beta}' \mathbf{Z}_{ij})]$ for $j = 1, 2, \ldots, N_i$. Thus, the joint survival function is

$$\Pr(X_{ij} > x_{ij}, j = 1, 2, \ldots, N_i | \mathbf{Z}_{ij}, j = 1, 2, \ldots, N_i)$$

$$= \varphi_\eta\left[\sum_{j=1}^{N_i} \varphi_\eta^{-1}\{\Pr(X_{ij} > x_{ij} | \mathbf{Z}_{ij})\} \right].$$

Examples of the Laplace transform and its inverse function are given in Table 2.1.

Table 2.1 Examples of frailty distributions

Distribution	Heterogeneity Parameter	Laplace: $\varphi_\eta(s)$	Inverse Laplace: $\varphi_\eta^{-1}(y)$	Kendall's tau: τ_η
Gamma	$\eta > 0$	$(1 + \eta s)^{-1/\eta}$	$(y^{-\eta} - 1)/\eta$	$\eta/(\eta + 2)$
Positive stable	$\eta \geq 0$	$\exp\{ -s^{1/(\eta+1)} \}$	$\{ -\log(y) \}^{\eta+1}$	$\eta/(\eta + 1)$
Log-normal	$\eta > 0$	Not available	Not available	Not available

For the gamma frailty model, one has $\varphi_\eta(s) = (1 + \eta s)^{-1/\eta}$ and $\varphi_\eta^{-1}(y) = (y^{-\eta} - 1)/\eta$. Thus,

$$\Pr(X_{ij} > x_{ij}, j = 1, 2, \ldots, N_{i0} | \mathbf{Z}_{ij}, j = 1, 2, \ldots, N_i)$$

$$= \left[\sum_{j=1}^{N_i} \Pr(X_{ij} > x_{ij} | \mathbf{Z}_{ij})^{-\eta} - (N_i - 1) \right]^{-\frac{1}{\eta}},$$

where the marginal distribution is $\Pr(X_{ij} > x_{ij} | \mathbf{Z}_{ij}) = [1 + \eta \Lambda_0(x_{ij}) \exp(\boldsymbol{\beta}' \mathbf{Z}_{ij})]^{-1/\eta}$. To investigate the correlation between X_{ij} and X_{ik} for $j \neq k$, we consider the bivariate survival function by letting $x_{ih} = 0$ for $h \neq j$ and $h \neq k$:

$$\Pr(X_{ij} > x_{ij}, X_{ik} > x_{ik} | \mathbf{Z}_{ij}, \mathbf{Z}_{ik})$$

$$= \left[\Pr(X_{ij} > x_{ij} | \mathbf{Z}_{ij})^{-\eta} + \Pr(X_{ik} > x_{ik} | \mathbf{Z}_{ik})^{-\eta} - 1 \right]^{-\frac{1}{\eta}}.$$

Kendall's tau (τ) is a measure of correlation between two random variables X_{ij} and X_{ik}. It can be shown in Sect. 2.6.1 that Kendall's tau is simply written as $\tau_{jk} =$

$\eta/(\eta + 2)$. Hence, a large value of η corresponds to a higher association, and $\eta = 0$ corresponds to independence.

The gamma frailty is the *conjugate* distribution for the Weibull distribution (Molenbergh et al. 2015). The resultant model is written as $\Pr(X_{ij} > x_{ij}|\mathbf{Z}_{ij}) = [1 + \eta\lambda x_{ij}^{\nu} \exp(\boldsymbol{\beta}'\mathbf{Z}_{ij})]^{-1/\eta}$ and called the Weibull–gamma distribution. The model is also known as the Burr-XII distribution (Burr 1942). The Weibull–gamma model permits the expression of mean and variance of X_{ij}.

2.5.2 Likelihood Function

We consider a dataset consisting of G independent clusters with the i-th cluster containing N_i patients. For $i = 1, 2, \ldots, G$ and $j = 1, 2, \ldots, N_i$, let

- X_{ij}: event time,
- C_{ij}: independent and non-informative censoring time.

The dataset consists of (T_{ij}, δ_{ij}, $\mathbf{Z}_{ij}$) for $i = 1, 2, \ldots, G$ and $j = 1, 2, \ldots, N_i$, where

- $T_{ij} = \min(X_{ij}, C_{ij})$: event time or censoring time whichever comes first,
- $\delta_{ij} = \mathbf{I}(T_{ij} = X_{ij})$: censoring status (censor = 0; event = 1),
  where $\mathbf{I}(\cdot)$ is the indicator function,
- $\mathbf{Z}_{ij}$: p-dimensional covariates.

Proposition 1 *Under the shared frailty model, the log-likelihood is*

$$\ell = \log L = \sum_{i=1}^{G} \left[\sum_{j=1}^{N_i} \delta_{ij} \log \lambda_{ij}(T_{ij}) \right.$$

$$\left. + \log \left\{ \int_{0}^{\infty} u_i^{m_i} \exp\left\{ -u_i \sum_{j=1}^{N_i} \Lambda_{ij}(T_{ij}) \right\} f_{\eta}(u_i)\mathrm{d}u_i \right\} \right].$$

where $\lambda_{ij}(t) = \lambda_0(t)\exp(\boldsymbol{\beta}'\mathbf{Z}_{ij})$, $\Lambda_{ij}(t) = \Lambda_0(t)\exp(\boldsymbol{\beta}'\mathbf{Z}_{ij})$, *and* $m_i = \sum_{j=1}^{N_i} \delta_{ij}$. *In particular, under the gamma frailty model, the log-likelihood is*

$$\ell = \sum_{i=1}^{G} \left[\sum_{j=1}^{N_i} \delta_{ij} \log \lambda_{ij}(T_{ij}) + m_i \log \eta + \log \Gamma\left(m_i + \frac{1}{\eta} \right) - \log \Gamma\left(\frac{1}{\eta} \right) \right.$$

$$\left. - \left(m_i + \frac{1}{\eta} \right) \log\left\{ 1 + \eta \sum_{j=1}^{N_i} \Lambda_{ij}(T_{ij}) \right\} \right].$$

Proof of Proposition 1: Define notations $\mathbf{T}_i = (T_{i1}, \ldots, T_{iN_i})$ and $\boldsymbol{\delta}_i = (\delta_{i1}, \cdots, \delta_{iN_i})$. Since the G clusters are independent, the likelihood takes the form $L = \prod_{i=1}^{G} L_i$, where L_i is the contribution from the i-th cluster. To compute L_i, we recall the assumptions:

- All patients in the i-th cluster share the common frailty term u_i,
- All patients in the i-th cluster are independent given the frailty term u_i,

Under these assumptions, L_i is computed as in Eq. (2.1) given u_i. Accordingly,

$$L_i(\mathbf{T}_i, \boldsymbol{\delta}_i | u_i) = \prod_{j=1}^{N_i} \{u_i \lambda_{ij}(T_{ij})\}^{\delta_{ij}} \exp\{-u_i \Lambda_{ij}(T_{ij})\}$$

$$= u_i^{m_i} \left\{ \prod_{j=1}^{N_i} \lambda_{ij}(T_{ij})^{\delta_{ij}} \right\} \exp\left\{ -u_i \sum_{j=1}^{N_i} \Lambda_{ij}(T_{ij}) \right\}.$$

Integrating out the unobserved frailty term,

$$L(\mathbf{T}_i, \boldsymbol{\delta}_i) = \int_0^\infty L_i(\mathbf{T}_i, \boldsymbol{\delta}_i | u_i) f_\eta(u_i) du_i = \left\{ \prod_{j=1}^{N_i} \lambda_{ij}(T_{ij})^{\delta_{ij}} \right\}$$

$$\times \int_0^\infty u_i^{m_i} \exp\left\{ -u_i \sum_{j=1}^{N_i} \Lambda_{ij}(T_{ij}) \right\} f_\eta(u_i) du_i.$$

Combining the likelihoods for the G independent clusters,

$$L = \prod_{i=1}^{G} L_i(\mathbf{T}_i, \ \boldsymbol{\delta}_i) = \prod_{i=1}^{G} \left[\left\{ \prod_{j=1}^{N_i} \lambda_{ij}(T_{ij})^{\delta_{ij}} \right\} \right.$$

$$\left. \times \int_0^\infty u_i^{m_i} \exp\left\{ -u_i \sum_{j=1}^{N_i} \Lambda_{ij}(T_{ij}) \right\} f_\eta(u_i) du_i \right].$$

The log-likelihood is obtained by taking the logarithm of the above expression. The log-likelihood under the gamma frailty model is obtained from the integral

$$\int_0^\infty u_i^{m_i} \exp\left\{ -u_i \sum_{j=1}^{N_i} \Lambda_{ij}(T_{ij}) \right\} f_\eta(u_i) du_i = \frac{\eta^{m_i} \Gamma(m_i + 1/\eta)}{\Gamma(1/\eta)}$$

■

$$\left(1 + \eta \sum_{j=1}^{N_i} \Lambda_{ij}(T_{ij}) \right)^{-m_i - 1/\eta}.$$

Many computing techniques and statistical packages for maximizing the log-likelihood have been developed under a semi-parametric model, where the form of $\lambda_0(\cdot)$ is unspecified (Hirsch and Wienke 2012). Vu and Knuiman (2002), Duchateau et al. (2002), Klein and Moeschberger (2003), and Duchateau and Janssen (2007) developed EM algorithms. Ha et al. (2017) regard u_i as parameters, leading to an iterative algorithm under a hierarchical likelihood. The algorithms in the R packages *survival* and *frailtypack* do not use EM algorithms. Majority of software packages use either the log-normal or gamma frailty distribution (Hirsch and Wienke 2012).

The Newton–Raphson algorithms are useful under parametric models, where the form of $\lambda_0(\cdot)$ is parametrically specified. For instance, the R function, *nlm()* or *optim()*, can maximize the log-likelihood by a Newton–Raphson type algorithm. Examples for parametric models include the Weibull, log-normal, Pareto and Gamma distributions. Among those, the Weibull model is the most common choice, which specifies the baseline hazard function as $\lambda_0(t; \mathbf{h}) = \lambda \nu t^{\nu-1}$, where $\mathbf{h} = (\lambda, \nu), \lambda > 0$ is a scale parameter and $\nu > 0$ a shape parameter. However, the Weibull model has only two parameters and is unlikely to capture the local changes of the hazard over the follow-up period.

2.5.3 Penalized Likelihood and Spline

Rondeau et al. (2003) developed the spline method to obtain a smooth estimate of $\lambda_0(\cdot)$ for clustered survival data. They specify the baseline hazard function as $\lambda_0(t; \mathbf{h}) = \sum_{\ell=1}^{L} h_\ell M_\ell(t)$, where h_ℓ's are positive parameters and $M_\ell(t)$'s are the M-spline basis functions. Rondeau et al. (2003) proposed estimates $(\hat{\mathbf{h}}, \hat{\boldsymbol{\beta}}, \hat{\eta})$ that maximize a penalized likelihood

$$\ell(\mathbf{h}, \boldsymbol{\beta}, \eta) - \kappa \int \ddot{\lambda}_0(t; \mathbf{h})^2 \mathrm{d}t,$$

where $\ell(\mathbf{h}, \boldsymbol{\beta}, \eta)$ is the log-likelihood in Proposition 1, $\ddot{\lambda}_0(t; \mathbf{h}) = d^2\lambda_0(t; \mathbf{h})/dt^2$, and $\kappa > 0$ is a *smoothing parameter*. The smoothing parameter controls the degrees of penalty on the roughness of the baseline hazard function. The estimates can be computed by applying the *frailtypack* R package (Rondeau and Gonzalez 2005).

2.6 Copulas for Bivariate Event Times

In medical studies, it is common to record two event times for each patient. For instance, a patient's medical records may have time-to-locoregional progression and time-to-distant metastasis. In the analysis of such bivariate survival data, the key element is an appropriate account for dependence between event times.

A *copula* can be used to link two event times by specifying their dependence structure[1]. Let X and Y be two event times, and $\mathbf{Z}_1$ and $\mathbf{Z}_2$ be associated covariates, respectively. Also let $S_X(x|\mathbf{Z}_1) = \Pr(X > x \mid \mathbf{Z}_1)$ and $S_Y(y|\mathbf{Z}_2) = \Pr(Y > y \mid \mathbf{Z}_2)$ be the marginal survival functions. Given $\mathbf{Z} = (\mathbf{Z}_1, \ \mathbf{Z}_2)$, we consider a bivariate survival function

$$\Pr(X > x, Y > y|\mathbf{Z}) = C_\theta\{S_X(x|\mathbf{Z}_1), S_Y(y|\mathbf{Z}_2)\}, \tag{2.2}$$

where a function C_θ is called *bivariate copula*[2] (Sklar 1959; Nelsen 2006) and a parameter θ describes the degree of dependence between X and Y. With this model, the dependence structure between X and Y is fully described by C_θ. The examples of bivariate copulas are listed below:

The independence copula:

$$C(u, v) = uv,$$

The Clayton copula (Clayton 1978):

$$C_\theta(u, v) = (u^{-\theta} + v^{-\theta} - 1)^{-1/\theta}, \quad \theta > 0,$$

The Gumbel copula (Gumbel 1960)**, also known as the Hougaard copula**:

$$C_\theta(u, v) = \exp\left[-\{(-\log u)^{\theta+1} + (-\log v)^{\theta+1}\}^{\frac{1}{\theta+1}}\right], \quad \theta \geq 0,$$

The Farlie–Gumbel–Morgenstern (FGM) copula (Morgenstern 1956):

$$C(u, v) = uv\{1 + \theta(1 - u)(1 - v)\}, \quad -1 \leq \theta \leq 1.$$

Any bivariate copula is a bivariate distribution function whose marginal distributions are the uniform distribution on [0,1]. Hence, one can consider a pair of random variables (U, V) such that $\Pr(U \leq u, \ V \leq v) = C_\theta(u, \ v)$. If one defines a pair of random variables (X, Y) by transformations $X = S_X^{-1}(U \ |\mathbf{Z}_1)$ and $Y = S_Y^{-1}(V \ |\mathbf{Z}_2)$, its distribution satisfies Eq. (2.2).

The Clayton and Gumbel copulas are derived from the gamma frailty and positive stable frailty models, respectively. However, the FGM copula cannot be derived as a frailty model.

---

[1]In general, a copula can be used to link more than two event times. We only consider a *bivariate copula* in this book.

[2]One may say "bivariate survival copula" or simply "survival copula" since the copula is applied to survival function in Eq. (2.2). See Nelsen (2006) for details.

Figure 2.3 gives the scatter plots for pairs (U, V) under the Clayton copula. The plots exhibit positive dependence between U and V, where the levels of dependence are different between $\theta = 2$ (Kendall's tau $= 0.5$) and $\theta = 8$ (Kendall's tau $= 0.8$).

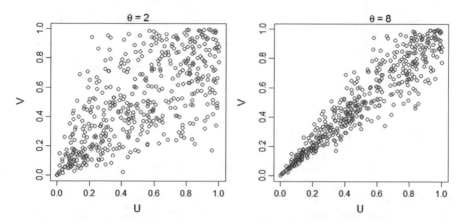

Fig. 2.3 The scatter plot for 500 pairs of (U, V) under the Clayton copula

The density function for C_θ is

$$C_\theta^{[1,1]}(u, v) = \frac{\partial^2}{\partial u \partial v} C_\theta(u, v), \quad 0 \le u \le 1, \quad 0 \le v \le 1.$$

Figure 2.4 gives the contour plots under the Clayton copula density. We see that the characteristic of the contour plots agrees with that for the scatter plots.

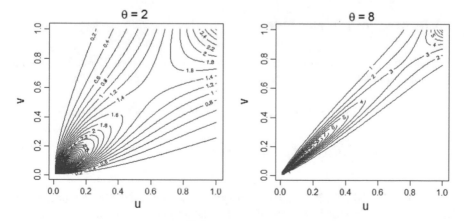

Fig. 2.4 The contour for the density $C_\theta^{[1,1]}(u, v)$ under the Clayton copula

Table 2.2 Examples of copulas

Copula	Parameter	Generator: $\phi_\theta(t)$	Kendall's tau: τ_θ	$r_\theta(s) = -s\ddot{\phi}_\theta(s)/\dot{\phi}_\theta(s)$
Independence	none	$-\log(t)$	0	1
Clayton	$\theta > 0$	$(t^{-\theta} - 1)/\theta$	$\theta/(\theta+2)$	$1+\theta$
Gumbel	$\theta \geq 0$	$\{-\log(t)\}^{\theta+1}$	$\theta/(\theta+1)$	$1-\theta/\log(s)$
FGM	$-1 \leq \theta \leq 1$	none	$2\theta/9$	none

An *Archimedean copula* is defined as

$$C_\theta(u, v) = \phi_\theta^{-1}\{\phi_\theta(u) + \phi_\theta(v)\},$$

where the function $\phi_\theta : [0, 1] \mapsto [0, \infty]$ is called a *generator* function of the copula, which is continuous and strictly decreasing from $\phi_\theta(0) > 0$ to $\phi_\theta(1) = 0$. Table 2.2 summarizes examples for generator functions. Any bivariate shared frailty model can be expressed as an Archimedean copula model by setting $\varphi_\eta^{-1}(t) = \phi_\eta(t)$. Hence, the copula models provide a more general framework of constructing bivariate survival models.

The Clayton copula has the generator $\phi_\theta(t) = (t^{-\theta} - 1)/\theta$ for $\theta > 0$. The limit $\lim_{\theta \to 0} \phi_\theta(t) = -\log(t)$ is also a generator for the independence copula. The FGM copula does not have a generator as it is not an Archimedean copula. In the Clayton, Gumbel, and FGM copulas, the value $\theta = 0$ reduces to the independence copula, namely, $\lim_{\theta \to 0} C_\theta(u, v) = uv$.

2.6.1 Measures of Dependence

Kendall's tau (τ) is a measure to assess the dependence between X and Y. It can be shown that Kendall's tau is solely expressed as a function of C_θ through

$$\tau_\theta = \Pr\{(X_1 - X_2)(Y_1 - Y_2) > 0\} - \Pr\{(X_1 - X_2)(Y_1 - Y_2) < 0\}$$

$$= 4 \int_0^1 \int_0^1 C_\theta(u, v) C_\theta^{[1,1]}(u, v) \mathrm{d}u \mathrm{d}v - 1, \tag{2.3}$$

where (X_1, Y_1) and (X_2, Y_2) are independently drawn from the copula model (2.2). This expression implies that Kendall's tau does not depend on how to specify the marginal survival functions $S_X(x|\mathbf{Z}_1) = \Pr(X > x \mid \mathbf{Z}_1)$ and $S_Y(y|\mathbf{Z}_2) = \Pr(Y > y \mid \mathbf{Z}_2)$.

An Archimedean copula has a "shortcut" formula to compute Kendall's tau

$$\tau_\theta = 1 + 4 \int_0^1 \frac{\phi_\theta(t)}{\dot{\phi}_\theta(t)} dt, \tag{2.4}$$

where $\dot{\phi}_\theta(t) = d\phi_\theta(t)/dt$. This formula gives $\tau_\theta = \theta/(\theta + 2)$ for the Clayton copula and $\tau_\theta = \theta/(\theta+1)$ for the Gumbel copula, both taking values from $\tau_0 = 0$ to $\tau_\infty = 1$.

Since the FGM copula is not an Archimedean copula, the shortcut formula cannot apply. However, the FGM copula has a simple expression $\tau_\theta = 2\theta/9$ for $-1 \leq \theta \leq 1$, which can be derived from Eq. (2.3). In the FGM copula, the range of Kendall's tau is restricted from $\tau_{-1} = -2/9$ to $\tau_1 = 2/9$.

It is convenient to define the partial derivatives of a copula:

$$C_\theta^{[1,0]}(u, v) = \frac{\partial}{\partial u} C_\theta(u, v), \quad C_\theta^{[0,1]}(u, v) = \frac{\partial}{\partial v} C_\theta(u, v),$$

$$C_\theta^{[1,1]}(u, v) = \frac{\partial^2}{\partial u \partial v} C_\theta(u, v).$$

Definition 7 The cross-ratio function (Oakes 1989) is defined as

$$R_\theta(u, v) = \frac{C_\theta^{[1,1]}(u, v) C_\theta(u, v)}{C_\theta^{[1,0]}(u, v) C_\theta^{[0,1]}(u, v)}.$$

The local dependence at a location (u, v) is defined as

- $R_\theta(u, v) > 1$; positive local dependence,
- $0 < R_\theta(u, v) < 1$; negative local dependence,
- $R_\theta(u, v) = 1$; local independence.

Under the independence copula, $R_\theta(u, v) = 1$ for $0 \leq u \leq 1$ and $0 \leq v \leq 1$. Remarkably, the Clayton copula has the constant cross-ratio $R_\theta(u, v) = 1 + \theta$.

A simplified formula of the cross-ratio function is available for an Archimedean copula. Using basic derivative rules, it can be shown that

$$R_\theta(u, v) = r_\theta\{C_\theta(u, v)\},$$

where $r_\theta(s) = -s\ddot{\phi}_\theta(s)/\dot{\phi}_\theta(s)$ and $\ddot{\phi}_\theta(t) = d^2\phi_\theta(t)/dt^2$. Table 2.2 shows the formulas for $r_\theta(\cdot)$ under selected copulas.

The cross-ratio function has a practical interpretation as the relative risk. Consider a medical follow-up in which the primary endpoint is OS, denoted as Y, and the secondary endpoint is TTP, denoted as X. We are interested in how tumour progression influences the risk of death. For this purpose, we consider the *conditional hazard functions*:

• $\lambda_Y(y|X = x, \mathbf{Z}) = \Pr(y \leq Y < y + dy|Y \geq y, X = x, \mathbf{Z})/dy$:

   – the hazard function of death given that a patient has experienced tumour progression at time x

• $\lambda_Y(y|X > x, \mathbf{Z}) = \Pr(y \leq Y < y + dy|Y \geq y, X > x, \mathbf{Z})/dy$:

   – the hazard function of death given that a patient has not yet experienced tumour progression at time x

Under a model $\Pr(X > x , Y > y|\mathbf{Z}) = C_\theta\{ S_X(x |\mathbf{Z}), S_Y(y |\mathbf{Z}) \}$, the relative risk is

$$\frac{\lambda_Y(y|X = x, \mathbf{Z})}{\lambda_Y(y|X > x, \mathbf{Z})} = R_\theta\{ S_X(x |\mathbf{Z}), S_Y(y |\mathbf{Z}) \}.$$

If $R_\theta > 1$, patients who have experienced tumour progression possess higher risk of death compared to those who have not yet. The Clayton copula yields the constant relative risk, and hence, is regarded as a type of proportional hazards models. In Chap. 5, we shall explore the role of the cross-ratio function on prognostic analysis under the joint frailty-copula model.

The cross-ratio function is also interpreted through the equation

$$\frac{\Pr(X = x, Y = y|\mathbf{Z}) \Pr(X > x, Y > y|\mathbf{Z})}{\Pr(X = x, Y > y|\mathbf{Z}) \Pr(X > x, Y = y|\mathbf{Z})} = R_\theta\{S_X(x|\mathbf{Z}), S_Y(y|\mathbf{Z})\}.$$

This is the odds ratio in the following 2×2 table (Table 2.3):

Table 2.3 A 2×2 table with the odds ratio AD/(BC)

	$Y = y$	$Y > y$
$X = x$	A	B
$X > x$	C	D

Clayton (1978) proposed to estimate θ by counting the number of events in each cell of the 2×2 tables, which is possible even when data are subject to right-censoring. Emura et al. (2010) generalized his idea to estimate θ under any member of Archimedean copulas by utilizing the formula $R_\theta(u, v) = r_\theta\{ C_\theta(u, v) \}$. See also Wang (2003), Emura and Wang (2010), and Emura et al. (2011) for the 2×2 table methods under Archimedean copula models.

We have seen that the Clayton copula has nice properties for statistical modeling: (i) a simple copula function, (ii) simple expression of Kendall's tau, (iii) constant cross-ratio function, and (iv) interpretability of the parameter $\theta + 1$ as the relative risk or odds ratio. These properties are useful for modeling bivariate survival data and interpreting the results of data analysis.

2.6.2 Residual Dependence

We shall introduce the concept of *residual dependence* between two endpoints. This type of dependence arises when covariates influencing two endpoints are ignored or missing.

Suppose that the primary endpoint is OS, denoted as Y, and the secondary endpoint is TTP, denoted as X. We impose the conditional independence between the two endpoints

$$\Pr(X > x, Y > y|\mathbf{Z}) = S_X(x|\mathbf{Z})S_Y(y|\mathbf{Z}), \tag{2.5}$$

where $S_X(x|\mathbf{Z}) = \Pr(X > x|\mathbf{Z})$ and $\Pr(Y > y|\mathbf{Z}) = S_Y(y|\mathbf{Z})$ are the marginal survival functions. If Eq. (2.5) holds, one can perform two separate Cox regression analyses for two endpoints. If Eq. (2.5) does not holds, the separate analyses may lose some information on dependence between endpoints and even produce biased results due to dependent censoring (Emura and Chen 2016, 2018).

To simplify our discussions, we consider a case, where only one covariate is measured. In this case, the conditional independence required for separate analyses is

$$\Pr(X > x, Y > y|Z_1) = S_X(x|Z_1)S_Y(y|Z_1),$$

where Z_1 is a covariate. However, the conditional independence typically does not hold for only one covariate Z_1. To see this, let $\mathbf{Z} = (Z_1, Z_2)$ be a two-dimensional vector of covariates that influence the two endpoints. Suppose that Z_2 is ignored as it is difficult to measure or is inconsistently measured (e.g., tumour volume). Figure 2.5 explains how the conditional independence fails to hold by omitting Z_2. Since Z_2 relates to the two endpoints, the variation in Z_2 induces unobserved frailty. For instance, a high (low) value of Z_2 is linked to short (long) values of X and Y. Consequently, X and Y exhibit positive association.

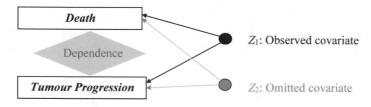

Fig. 2.5 Residual dependence between death and tumour progression

The above discussions lead to a principle that the conditional independence is less likely to hold if many important covariates are omitted or ignored from the model. This mechanism of yielding dependence is termed *residual dependence*. Residual dependence arises in a meta-analysis where important covariates are missing in some studies (Chap. 3; Emura et al. 2017). In this case, the copula model (2.2) can help relax the conditional independence.

2.6.3 Likelihood Function

We consider *bivariate survival data* containing N patients. For $j = 1, 2, \ldots, N$, let

- (X_j, Y_j): a pair of event times,
- (C_j, C_j^*): a pair of censoring times for (X_j, Y_j),

Bivariate survival data consist of $\{(T_j, T_j^*, \delta_j, \delta_j^*, \mathbf{Z}_j); j = 1, 2, \ldots, N\}$, where $T_j = \min(X_j, C_j)$, $T_j^* = \min(Y_j, C_j^*)$, $\delta_j = \mathbf{I}(T_j = X_j)$, $\delta_j^* = \mathbf{I}(T_j^* = Y_j)$, and $\mathbf{Z}_j = (\mathbf{Z}_{1j}, \mathbf{Z}_{2j})$ is a vector of covariates.

Proposition 2 *Under the copula model* $\Pr(X > x, Y > y|\mathbf{Z}) = C_\theta\{S_X(x|\mathbf{Z}_1), S_Y(y|\mathbf{Z}_2)\}$, *the log-likelihood is*

$$\ell = \log L = \sum_{j=1}^{n} \Big[\delta_j \log \lambda_X(T_j|\mathbf{Z}_{1j}) + \delta_j^* \log \lambda_Y(T_j^*|\mathbf{Z}_{2j})$$
$$+ \delta_j \delta_j^* \log R_\theta\{S_X(T_j|\mathbf{Z}_{1j}), S_Y(T_j^*|\mathbf{Z}_{2j})\}$$
$$+ \delta_j \log \eta_{1,\theta}\{S_X(T_j|\mathbf{Z}_{1j}), S_Y(T_j^*|\mathbf{Z}_{2j})\}$$
$$+ \delta_j^* \log \eta_{2,\theta}\{S_X(T_j|\mathbf{Z}_{1j}), S_Y(T_j^*|\mathbf{Z}_{2j})\}$$
$$+ \log C_\theta\{S_X(T_j|\mathbf{Z}_{1j}), S_Y(T_j^*|\mathbf{Z}_{2j})\}\Big].$$

where $\lambda_X(t|\mathbf{Z}_{1j}) = -\partial \log S_X(t|\mathbf{Z}_{1j})/\partial t$, $\lambda_Y(t|\mathbf{Z}_{2j}) = -\partial \log S_Y(t|\mathbf{Z}_{2j})/\partial t$, $\eta_{\theta,1}(u, v) = u \frac{C_\theta^{[1,0]}(u, v)}{C_\theta(u, v)}$ *and* $\eta_{2,\theta}(u, v) = v \frac{C_\theta^{[0,1]}(u, v)}{C_\theta(u, v)}$.

Proof of Proposition 2: Each patient experiences one of the four cases: (i) $\delta_j = \delta_j^* = 1$, (ii) $\delta_j = 1$ and $\delta_j^* = 0$, (iii) $\delta_j = 0$ and $\delta_j^* = 1$, and (iv) $\delta_j = \delta_j^* = 0$. Each case has its own likelihood. Combining the four cases, the likelihood for the j-th patient is

$$L_j = \Pr(X_j = T_j, Y_j = T_j^*|\mathbf{Z}_j)^{\delta_j \delta_j^*} \Pr(X_j = T_j, Y_j > T_j^*|\mathbf{Z}_j)^{\delta_j(1-\delta_j^*)}$$
$$\times \Pr(X_j > T_j, Y_j = T_j^*|\mathbf{Z}_j)^{(1-\delta_j)\delta_j^*} \Pr(X_j > T_j, Y_j > T_j^*|\mathbf{Z}_j)^{(1-\delta_j)(1-\delta_j^*)}$$

$$= \left\{ \frac{\Pr(X_j = T_j, Y_j = T_j^* | \mathbf{Z}_j) \Pr(X_j > T_j, Y_j > T_j^* | \mathbf{Z}_j)}{\Pr(X_j = T_j, Y_j > T_j^* | \mathbf{Z}_j) \Pr(X_j > T_j, Y_j = T_j^* | \mathbf{Z}_j)} \right\}^{\delta_j \delta_j^*}$$

$$\times \left\{ \frac{\Pr(X_j = T_j, Y_j > T_j^* | \mathbf{Z}_j)}{\Pr(X_j > T_j, Y_j > T_j^* | \mathbf{Z}_j)} \right\}^{\delta_j} \left\{ \frac{\Pr(X_j > T_j, Y_j = T_j^* | \mathbf{Z}_j)}{\Pr(X_j > T_j, Y_j > T_j^* | \mathbf{Z}_j)} \right\}^{\delta_j^*}$$

$$\times \Pr(X_j > T_j, Y_j > T_j^* | \mathbf{Z}_j).$$

Under the copula model,

$$L_j = R_\theta \{ S_X(T_j | \mathbf{Z}_{1j}), S_Y(T_j^* | \mathbf{Z}_{2j}) \}^{\delta_j \delta_j^*}$$

$$\left[-\frac{\partial}{\partial T_j} S_X(T_j | \mathbf{Z}_{1j}) \frac{C_\theta^{[1,0]} \{ S_X(T_j \mathbf{Z}_{1j}), S_Y(T_j^* | \mathbf{Z}_{2j}) \}}{C_\theta \{ S_X(T_j | \mathbf{Z}_{1j}), S_Y(T_j^* | \mathbf{Z}_{2j}) \}} \right]^{\delta_j}$$

$$\times \left[-\frac{\partial}{\partial T_j^*} S_Y(T_j^* | \mathbf{Z}_{2j}) \frac{C_\theta^{[0,1]} \{ S_X(T_j | \mathbf{Z}_{1j}), S_Y(T_j^* | \mathbf{Z}_{2j}) \}}{C_\theta \{ S_X(T_j | \mathbf{Z}_{1j}), S_Y(T_j^* | \mathbf{Z}_{2j}) \}} \right]^{\delta_j^*}$$

$$C_\theta \{ S_X(T_j | \mathbf{Z}_{1j}), S_Y(T_j^* | \mathbf{Z}_{2j}) \}$$

$$= \lambda_X(T_j | \mathbf{Z}_{1j})^{\delta_j} \times \lambda_Y(T_j^* | \mathbf{Z}_{2j})^{\delta_j^*} R_\theta \{ S_X(T_j | \mathbf{Z}_{1j}), S_Y(T_j^* | \mathbf{Z}_{2j}) \}^{\delta_j \delta_j^*}$$

$$\times \left[\eta_{\theta,1} \{ S_X(T_j | \mathbf{Z}_{1j}), S_Y(T_j^* | \mathbf{Z}_{2j}) \} \right]^{\delta_j} \left[\eta_{\theta,2} \{ S_X(T_j | \mathbf{Z}_{1j}), S_Y(T_j^* | \mathbf{Z}_{2j}) \} \right]^{\delta_j^*}$$

$$\times C_\theta \{ S_X(T_j | \mathbf{Z}_{1j}), S_Y(T_j^* | \mathbf{Z}_{2j}) \}.$$

The log-likelihood is obtained by taking the logarithm of the above expression. ∎

The likelihood-based procedures developed in Sect. 2.4 are applicable to the likelihood function in Proposition 2. The following proposition follows since $R_\theta(u, v) = \eta_{\theta,1}(u, v) = \eta_{\theta,1}(u, v) = 1$ under $C_\theta(u, v) = uv$.

Proposition 3 *Under the independence model* $\Pr(X > x, Y > y | \mathbf{Z}) = S_X(x | \mathbf{Z}_1) \times S_Y(y | \mathbf{Z}_2)$, *the log-likelihood is* $\ell = \ell_X + \ell_Y$, *where*

$$\ell_X = \sum_{j=1}^{n} [\delta_j \log \lambda_X(T_j | \mathbf{Z}_{1j}) - \Lambda_X(T_j | \mathbf{Z}_{1j})],$$

$$\ell_Y = \sum_{j=1}^{n} [\delta_j^* \log \lambda_Y(T_j^* | \mathbf{Z}_{2j}) - \Lambda_Y(T_j^* | \mathbf{Z}_{2j})],$$

where $\Lambda_X(t | \mathbf{Z}_{1j}) = -\log S_X(t | \mathbf{Z}_{1j})$ *and* $\Lambda_Y(t | \mathbf{Z}_{2j}) = -\log S_Y(t | \mathbf{Z}_{2j})$.

Proposition 3 implies that, under the independence model, one can obtains the MLE by maximizing ℓ_X based on data $\{(T_j, \delta_j, \mathbf{Z}_{1j}); j = 1, 2, \ldots, N\}$ and maximizing ℓ_Y based on data $\{(T_j^*, \delta_j^*, \mathbf{Z}_{2j}); j = 1, 2, \ldots, N\}$ as discussed in Sect. 2.4. However, the two separate analyses yield inefficient estimators due to the loss caused by ignoring dependence between two event times.

2.7 Exercises

1. Is TTP an adequate endpoint in advanced colorectal cancer? After reading Chapter 2 and Piedbois and Croswell (2008), please write a one-page report to summarize your answers.
2. Are the following statements correct? Please verify your answers.

   (1) PFS $\leq$ OS holds for all patients in a clinical trial.
   (2) TTP $\leq$ OS holds for all patients in a clinical trial.
   (3) PFS $\leq$ TTP holds for all patients in a clinical trial.
   (4) PFS $<$ OS holds for all patients in a clinical trial.

3. Answer the following questions by performing Cox regression on the 63 training samples from the lung cancer data available in the *compound.Cox* R package (Emura et al. 2019).

   (1) Is *ZNF264* univariately associated with survival (P-value < 0.05)?
   (2) Is *NF1* univariately associated with survival (P-value < 0.05)?
   (3) Are *ZNF264* and *NF1* associated with survival (P-value < 0.05)?
   (4) Discuss about the multicollinearity between *ZNF264* and *NF1*.
   (5) How many genes are univariately associated with survival (P-value < 0.05)?

4. We analyze the data (T_i, δ_i, Z_i), $i = 1, \ldots, n$, under the model $S(t|Z_i) = \exp\{-\lambda t \exp(\beta Z_i)\}$, where $\lambda > 0$, $-\infty < \beta < \infty$, and $Z_i = 0$ or 1. Let $m = \sum_{i=1}^{n} \delta_i$, $n_1 = \sum_{i=1}^{n} Z_i$, and $n_0 = n - n_1$.

   (1) Write down the log-likelihood function $\ell(\boldsymbol{\varphi})$, where $\boldsymbol{\varphi} = (\lambda, \beta)$.
   (2) Obtain the MLE by solving the score equation $\mathbf{S}(\boldsymbol{\varphi}) = \mathbf{0}$.
   (3) Derive the Hessian matrix of $H(\boldsymbol{\varphi}) = \partial^2 \ell(\boldsymbol{\varphi})/\partial\boldsymbol{\varphi}\partial\boldsymbol{\varphi}'$.
   (4) Derive the Newton–Raphson algorithm and apply it to the data of Sect. 2.3.1.
   (5) Compare the estimate $\exp(\hat{\beta})$ with the one obtained from the partial likelihood.

5. Derive the mean $E[X|\ \mathbf{Z}]$ and variance $Var(X|\ \mathbf{Z})$ for the Weibull–gamma distribution $\Pr(X > x|\mathbf{Z}) = [1 + \eta\lambda x^\nu \exp(\boldsymbol{\beta}'\mathbf{Z})]^{-1/\eta}$.
6. Consider a Gamma(α, β) distribution with the density

$$ f_{\alpha,\beta}(u) = \frac{1}{\Gamma(\alpha)\beta^\alpha} u^{\alpha-1} \exp\left(-\frac{u}{\beta}\right), \quad \alpha > 0, \quad \beta > 0, \quad u > 0. $$

   (1) Show $E(\ \log u\ ) = \psi(\alpha) + \log\beta$, where $\psi(\alpha) = d\{\log\Gamma(\alpha)\}/d\alpha$ is the digamma function.

(2) Under Gamma($\alpha = 1/\eta$, $\beta = \eta$), derive the conditional distribution

$$(u_i | \mathbf{T}_i, \delta_i) \sim \text{Gamma}\left(\alpha = \frac{1}{\eta} + m_i, \beta = \left\{\frac{1}{\eta} + \sum_{j=1}^{N_i} \Lambda_{ij}(T_{ij})\right\}^{-1}\right).$$

Hint: $f(u_i | \mathbf{T}_i, \delta_i) \propto L_i(\mathbf{T}_i, \delta_i | u_i) f(u_i)$, where $L_i(\mathbf{T}_i, \delta_i | u_i)$ is in the proof of Proposition 1.

(3) Show

$$E(u_i | \mathbf{T}_i, \delta_i) = \frac{1/\eta + m_i}{1/\eta + \sum_{j=1}^{N_i} \Lambda_{ij}(T_{ij})},$$

$$E(\log u_i | \mathbf{T}_i, \delta_i) = \psi\left(\frac{1}{\eta} + m_i\right) - \log\left\{\frac{1}{\eta} + \sum_{j=1}^{N_i} \Lambda_{ij}(T_{ij})\right\}.$$

7. Under the FGM copula, derive the expression of Kendall's tau $\tau_\theta = 2\theta/9$ for $-1 \le \theta \le 1$.
8. Under the Clayton copula and Gumbel copula, derive the expressions of Kendall's tau $\tau_\theta = \theta/(\theta + 2)$ and $\tau_\theta = \theta/(\theta + 1)$, respectively.
9. We consider the log-likelihood of Proposition 2 under the Clayton copula.

   (1) Derive the forms of $\eta_{\theta,1}(u, v)$, $\eta_{2,\theta}(u, v)$, and $R_\theta(u, v)$.
   (2) Write down the log-likelihood.

References

Andersen PK, Borgan O, Gill RD, Keiding N (1993) Statistical models based on counting processes. Springer-Verlag, New York

Burr IW (1942) Cumulative frequency functions. Ann Math Stat 13(2):215–232

Cheema PK, Burkes RL (2013). Overall survival should be the primary endpoint in clinical trials for advanced non-small-cell lung cancer. Curr Oncol 20:e150–160

Clayton DG (1978) A model for association in bivariate life tables and its application in epidemiological studies of familial tendency in chronic disease incidence. Biometrika 65(1):141–151

Cox DR (1972) Regression models and life-tables (with discussion). J R Stat Soc Series B Stat Methodol 34:187–220

Duchateau L, Janssen P, Lindsey P, Legrand C, Nguti R, Sylvester R (2002) The shared frailty model and the power for heterogeneity tests in multicenter trials. Comput Stat Data Anal 40(3):603–620

Duchateau L, Janssen P (2007) The frailty model. Springer, New York

Eisenhauer E, Therasse P, Bogaerts J, et al (2009) New response evaluation criteria in solid tumours: revised RECIST guideline (version 1.1). Eur J Cancer 45(2):228–247

Emura T (2019) joint.Cox: joint frailty-copula models for tumour progression and death in meta-analysis, CRAN

Emura T, Chen YH (2016) Gene selection for survival data under dependent censoring, a copula-based approach. Stat Methods Med Res 25(6):2840–2857

Emura T, Chen YH (2018). Analysis of survival data with dependent censoring, copula-based approaches, JSS Research Series in Statistics. Springer

Emura T, Matsui S, Chen HY (2019) compound.Cox: univariate feature selection and compound covariate for predicting survival. Comput Methods Programs Biomed 168:21–37

Emura T, Lin CW, Wang W (2010) A goodness-of-fit test for Archimedean copula models in the presence of right censoring. Compt Stat Data Anal 54:3033–3043

Emura T, Nakatochi M, Murotani K, Rondeau V (2017) A joint frailty-copula model between tumour progression and death for meta-analysis. Stat Methods Med Res 26(6):2649–2666

Emura T, Nakatochi M, Matsui S, Michimae H, Rondeau V (2018) Personalized dynamic prediction of death according to tumour progression and high-dimensional genetic factors: meta-analysis with a joint model. Stat Methods Med Res 27(9):2842–2858

Emura T, Wang W (2010) Testing quasi-independence for truncation data. J Multivar Anal 101:223–239

Emura T, Wang W, Hung HN (2011) Semi-parametric inference for copula models for dependently truncated data. Stat Sinica 21:349–367

Fleming TR, Harrington DP (1991). Counting processes and survival analysis. Wiley, USA

Ganzfried BF, Riester M, Haibe-Kains B, et al (2013) Curated ovarian data: clinically annotated data for the ovarian cancer transcriptome, Database; Article ID bat013. https://doi.org/10.1093/database/bat013

Green EM, Yothers G, Sargent DJ (2008) Surrogate endpoint validation: statistical elegance versus clinical relevance. Stat Methods Med Res 17(5):477–486

Gumbel EJ (I960). Distributions de valeurs extremes en plusieurs dimensions. PubL Inst Statist. Parids 9:171–173

Ha ID, Jeong JH, Lee Y (2017) Statistical modelling of survival data with random effects: h-likelihood approach. Springer, Singapore

Hamasaki T, Asakura K, Evans SR, Ochiai T (2016) Group-sequential clinical trials with multiple co-objectives. JSS Series in Statistics. Springer, New York

Hirsch K, Wienke A (2012) Software for semiparametric shared gamma and log-normal frailty models: an overview. Comput Methods Programs Biomed 107(3):582–597

Kalbfleisch JD, Prentice RL (2002) The statistical analysis of failure time data, 2nd edn. Wiley, New York

Klein JP, Moeschberger ML (2003) Survival analysis techniques for censored and truncated data. Springer, New York

Le Tourneau C, Michiels S, Gan HK, Siu LL (2009) Reporting of time-to-event end points and tracking of failures in randomized trials of radiotherapy with or without any concomitant anticancer agent for locally advanced head and neck cancer. J Clin Oncol 27(35):5965–5971

Matsui S, Buyse M, Simon R (eds) (2015) Design and analysis of clinical trials for predictive medicine, vol 72. CRC Press, New York

Michiels S, Le Maître A, Buyse M, Burzykowski T, Maillard E, Bogaerts J, Pignon JP (2009) Surrogate endpoints for overall survival in locally advanced head and neck cancer: meta-analyses of individual patient data. Lancet Oncol 10(4):341–350

Molenberghs G, Verbeke G, Efendi A, Braekers R, Demétrio CG (2015) A combined gamma frailty and normal random-effects model for repeated, overdispersed time-to-event data. Stat Methods Med Res 24(4):434–452

Morgenstern D (1956) Einfache Beispiele zweidimensionaler Verteilungen. Mitteilungsblatt für Mathematishe Statistik. 8:234–235

Nelsen RB (2006) An introduction to copulas, 2nd edn. Springer, New York

Oakes D (1989) Bivariate survival models induced by frailties. J Am Stat Assoc 84:487–493

Oba K, Paoletti X, Alberts S et al (2013) Disease-free survival as a surrogate for overall survival in adjuvant trials of gastric cancer: a meta-analysis. J Natl Cancer Inst 105(21):1600–1607

Pazdur R (2008) Endpoints for assessing drug activity in clinical trials. Oncologist 13:19–21

Piedbois P, Croswell MJ (2008) Surrogate endpoints for overall survival in advanced colorectal cancer: a clinician's perspective. Stat Methods Med Res 17(5):519–527

Ramsay J (1988) Monotone regression spline in action. Statis Sci 3:425–461

Rodríguez-Girondo M, Deelen J, Slagboom EP, Houwing-Duistermaat JJ (2018) Survival analysis with delayed entry in selected families with application to human longevity. Stat Methods Med Res 27(3):933–954

Rondeau V, Commenges D, Joly P (2003) Maximum penalized likelihood estimation in a gamma-frailty model. Lifetime Data Anal 9:139–153

Rondeau V, Gonzalez JR (2005) frailtypack: a computer program for the analysis of correlated failure time data using penalized likelihood estimation. Comput Methods Programs Biomed 80(2):154–164

Rondeau V, Pignon JP, Michiels S (2015) A joint model for dependence between clustered times to tumour progression and deaths: a meta-analysis of chemotherapy in head and neck cancer. Stat Methods Med Res 24(6):711–729

Rondeau V, Mauguen A, Laurent A, Berr C, Helmer C (2017) Dynamic prediction models for clustered and interval-censored outcomes: investigating the intra-couple correlation in the risk of dementia. Stat Methods Med Res 26(5):2168–2183

Shi Q, Sargent DJ (2009) Meta-analysis for the evaluation of surrogate endpoints in cancer clinical trials. Int J Clin Oncol 14(2):102–111

Sklar A (1959) Fonctions de répartition à n dimensions et leurs marges. Publications de l'Institut de Statistique de L'Université de Paris. 8:229–231

Soria JC, Massard C, Le Chevalier T (2010) Should progression-free survival be the primary measure of efficacy for advanced NSCLC therapy? Ann Oncol 21(12):2324–2332

Sugimoto T, Hamasaki T, Evans SR (2017) Sizing clinical trials when comparing bivariate time-to-event outcomes. Stat Med 36(9):1363–1382

Vu HT, Knuiman MW (2002) A hybrid ML-EM algorithm for calculation of maximum likelihood estimates in semiparametric shared frailty models. Compt Stat Data Anal 40(1):173–187

Wang W (2003) Estimating the association parameter for copula models under dependent censoring. J R Stat Soc Series B Stat Methodol 65(1):257–273

Chapter 3
The Joint Frailty-Copula Model for Correlated Endpoints

Abstract This chapter describes a meta-analysis (or multicenter analysis) of individual patient data with two correlated survival endpoints. The endpoints of interest are time-to-tumour progression (TTP) and overall survival (OS). We first define a semi-competing risks setting for TTP and OS. We then introduce the *joint frailty-copula model* that formulates the shared frailty model for heterogeneity in a meta-analysis, and utilizes a copula for dependence between TTP and OS. To account for the effect that TTP is dependently censored by death, a likelihood function is derived under the semi-competing risks setting. We adopt spline-based models for baseline hazard functions with the aid of a penalized likelihood procedure. We analyze the data on ovarian cancer patients to illustrate statistical analyses using the *joint.Cox* R package.

Keywords Clayton's copula · Cox regression · Individual-level dependence · Penalized likelihood · Residual dependence · Semi-competing risk · Spline · Surrogate endpoint

3.1 Introduction

We consider a meta-analysis to perform Cox regression for both time-to-tumour progression (TTP) and overall survival (OS). In this respect, Burzykowski et al. (2001) developed a bivariate Weibull model for jointly performing Cox regression for two endpoints with meta-analytic data. See also Chap. 11 of Burzykowski et al. (2005). They proposed a two-step method; the first step applies a copula to account for the individual-level dependence between two endpoints, and the second stage applies random-effects to account for heterogeneity in a meta-analysis. The two-step method of Burzykowski et al. (2001, 2005) has been applied to a number of cancer studies for evaluating the correlations of two endpoints and is recently implemented in an R package (Rotolo et al. 2018).

© The Author(s), under exclusive license to Springer Nature Singapore Pte Ltd. 2019
T. Emura et al., *Survival Analysis with Correlated Endpoints*,
JSS Research Series in Statistics, https://doi.org/10.1007/978-981-13-3516-7_3

While the two-step method can account for dependence between two endpoints through a copula, the estimation method cannot account for the effect of dependent censoring. In other words, the two-step method is valid only when two endpoints are subject to independent censoring. There would be a concern for bias when we assess TTP through the two-step method since TTP is *dependently* censored by death. Since death may be highly associated with tumour progression, censoring due to death is less likely to be independent.

Statistical methods for semi-competing risks data properly deal with the case where death can dependently censor TTP (Fine et al. 2001). This setting regards death as a competing risk for TTP rather than treating death as an independent censoring for TTP (Haneuse and Lee 2016). Under the semi-competing risks setup, Rondeau et al. (2015) developed a one-step estimation method based on a joint frailty model, where a frailty term account for heterogeneity in a meta-analysis. The joint frailty model can induce the intra-study dependence between TTP and OS through unobserved frailties. However, there exists some residual dependence (individual-level dependence) in meta-analyses (Burzykowski et al. 2001, 2005). Emura et al. (2017) extended the joint frailty model of Rondeau et al. (2015) to account for the residual dependence via copulas, after having accounted for the intra-study dependency with frailties. While their copula model is similar to that of Burzykowski et al. (2001), the estimation procedure of Emura et al. (2017) incorporates the effect of dependent censoring (semi-competing risk) into the likelihood. In addition, their approach adopts cubic splines for the baseline hazard functions, providing more flexible models over the Weibull model of Burzykowski et al. (2001) and Rotolo et al. (2018). Under the copula models, Peng et al. (2018) developed an even more flexible model, where the forms of the baseline hazard functions are completely unspecified.

In the sequel, we introduce the estimation procedure of Emura et al. (2017) and its implementation via the *joint.Cox* R package (Emura 2019).

3.2 Semi-competing Risks Data

Meta-analysis using patient-level information is called *individual patient data* (IPD) meta-analysis. IPD meta-analysis is essentially different from meta-analysis on summary data or published data where patient-level information is lost. We only consider IPD meta-analyses since patient-level information is required to assess dependence between endpoints.

We consider an IPD meta-analysis on data consisting of G independent studies with the ith study containing N_i patients. For $i = 1, 2, \ldots, G$ and $j = 1, 2, \ldots, N_i$, let

- X_{ij}: time-to-tumour progression (TTP),
- D_{ij}: overall survival (OS), or equivalently time-to-death,
- C_{ij}: independent and noninformative censoring time.

Figure 3.1 provides observation patterns of data where each patient exhibits one of the four mutually exclusive cases (Cases A–D). First, if a patient experiences tumour progression and then dies before independent censoring time, both TTP and OS are available (Case A). Second, if a patient experiences tumour progression but does not die before independent censoring time, then TTP is available but OS is censored (Case B). Third, if a patient dies without tumour progression, then OS is available, but TTP is dependently censored by death (Case C). Fourth, if a patient experiences neither tumour progression nor death before independent censoring time, both TTP and OS are censored (Case D).

Consequently, what we actually observe can be written as $(T_{ij}, T_{ij}^*, \delta_{ij}, \delta_{ij}^*, \mathbf{Z}_{1,ij}, \mathbf{Z}_{2,ij})$ for $i = 1, 2, \ldots, G$ and $j = 1, 2, \ldots, N_i$, where

- $T_{ij} = \min(X_{ij}, D_{ij}, C_{ij})$: first-occurring event time,
- $\delta_{ij} = \mathbf{I}(T_{ij} = X_{ij})$: status of tumour progression (no progression = 0; progression = 1),
  where $\mathbf{I}(\cdot)$ is the indicator function,
- $T_{ij}^* = \min(D_{ij}, C_{ij})$: censored terminal event time,
- $\delta_{ij}^* = \mathbf{I}(T_{ij}^* = D_{ij})$: vital status (alive = 0; dead = 1),
- $\mathbf{Z}_{1,ij}$: p_1-dimensional covariates associated with TTP,
- $\mathbf{Z}_{2,ij}$: p_2-dimensional covariates associated with OS.

The four cases (Cases A–D in Fig. 3.1) can be identified by a pair $(\delta_{ij}, \delta_{ij}^*)$. For instance, Case A corresponds to the pair $(\delta_{ij}, \delta_{ij}^*) = (1, 1)$ whereby $T_{ij} = X_{ij}$ and $T_{ij}^* = D_{ij}$. Table 3.1 summarized the four possible pairs, $(\delta_{ij}, \delta_{ij}^*) = (1, 1), (1, 0), (0, 1)$, and $(0, 0)$.

The aforementioned observation patterns follow the *semi-competing risks* setting (Fine et al. 2001) in which *terminal event* is a competing risk for *nonterminal event*. In our setting, death (terminal event) can dependently censor TTP (nonterminal event); see Case C in Fig. 3.1. On the other hand, tumour progression cannot censor OS; see Case A in Fig. 3.1. Hence, death is a competing risk for tumour progression, but tumor progression is not a competing risk for death, suggesting the term "semi-competing risks". The censoring of TTP by death is termed *dependent censoring* that is distinguished from the usual *independent censoring*. What we defined as TTP can actually be any nonterminal event such as "time-to-recurrence".

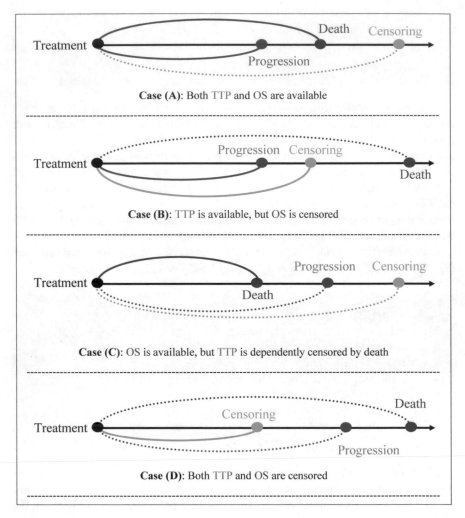

Fig. 3.1 Observation patters of semi-competing risks data. Observed event times are denoted by solid lines and unobserved event times are denoted by dotted lines

Table 3.1 Observation patterns of semi-competing risks data

	First event	Last event	T_{ij}	T_{ij}^*	δ_{ij}	δ_{ij}^*
Case (A)	Tumour progression	Death	X_{ij}	D_{ij}	1	1
Case (B)	Tumour progression	Independent censoring	X_{ij}	C_{ij}	1	0
Case (C)	Death	Death	D_{ij}	D_{ij}	0	1
Case (D)	Independent censoring	Independent censoring	C_{ij}	C_{ij}	0	0

3.3 Joint Frailty-Copula Model

It is generally understood that meta-analyses should assess heterogeneity between studies. Hence, an appropriate model for meta-analysis may include a study specific (random) effect to account for heterogeneity. To capture the heterogeneity of baseline risks, Rondeau et al. (2015) considered unobserved frailty terms $u_i(i = 1, 2, \ldots, G)$, which act on the hazard functions for TTP and OS. The frailty terms are assumed to follow a gamma distribution with a density

$$f_\eta(u) = \frac{1}{\Gamma(1/\eta)\eta^{1/\eta}} u^{\frac{1}{\eta}-1} \exp\left(-\frac{u}{\eta}\right), \quad u > 0, \quad \eta > 0.$$

The distribution has mean 1 and variance η that represents the degree of the between-study heterogeneity. Conditional on u_i, $\mathbf{Z}_{1,ij}$ and $\mathbf{Z}_{2,ij}$, we define the hazard functions

$$\begin{cases} r_{ij}(t|u_i) = \Pr(t \leq X_{ij} < t + dt | X_{ij} \geq t, u_i, \mathbf{Z}_{1,ij})/dt, \\ \lambda_{ij}(t|u_i) = \Pr(t \leq D_{ij} < t + dt | D_{ij} \geq t, u_i, \mathbf{Z}_{2,ij})/dt, \end{cases}$$

where $\mathbf{Z}_{1,ij}$ and $\mathbf{Z}_{2,ij}$ are suppressed on the left-hand sides. Rondeau et al. (2015) proposed a *joint frailty model* for meta-analysis:

Definition 1 The joint frailty model is defined as

$$\begin{cases} r_{ij}(t|u_i) = u_i r_0(t) \exp(\boldsymbol{\beta}_1' \mathbf{Z}_{1,ij}), \\ \lambda_{ij}(t|u_i) = u_i^\alpha \lambda_0(t) \exp(\boldsymbol{\beta}_2' \mathbf{Z}_{2,ij}). \end{cases} \tag{3.1}$$

In this model, X_{ij} and D_{ij} are assumed to be conditionally independent given u_i, $\mathbf{Z}_{1,ij}$, and $\mathbf{Z}_{2,ij}$.

The parameters $\boldsymbol{\beta}_1$ (or $\boldsymbol{\beta}_2$) are the effects of $\mathbf{Z}_{1,ij}$(or $\mathbf{Z}_{2,ij}$), which are the target population parameters. The forms of the baseline hazard functions $r_0(\cdot)$ and $\lambda_0(\cdot)$ are flexibly modeled. Since the frailty term u_i is shared by the two hazard functions, it induces the intra-study dependence between X_{ij} and D_{ij}. The parameter α can differentiate the effect of heterogeneity between the two endpoints.

Residual dependence arises if a patient-level characteristics affecting both X_{ij} and D_{ij} is ignored in the model (Sect. 2.6.2). In meta-analysis, residual dependence is a legitimate concern since researchers often have a limited access to covariates. Emura et al. (2017) proposed a joint frailty-copula model that extends the joint frailty model by introducing the intra-subject dependence using a copula (Nelsen 2006):

Definition 2 The joint frailty-copula model is defined as

$$
\begin{cases}
r_{ij}(t|u_i) = u_i r_0(t) \exp(\boldsymbol{\beta}_1' \mathbf{Z}_{1,ij}) \\
\lambda_{ij}(t|u_i) = u_i^\alpha \lambda_0(t) \exp(\boldsymbol{\beta}_2' \mathbf{Z}_{2,ij}) \\
\Pr(X_{ij} > x, D_{ij} > y|u_i) = C_\theta[S_{Xij}(x|u_i), S_{Dij}(y|u_i)]
\end{cases}, \tag{3.2}
$$

where C_θ is a copula with an unknown parameter θ.

In Definition 2, the survival functions and hazard functions are related through

$$
\begin{cases}
S_{Xij}(x|u_i) = \exp\{-u_i R_0(x) \exp(\boldsymbol{\beta}_1' \mathbf{Z}_{1,ij})\}, & R_0(x) = \int_0^x r_0(t)\mathrm{d}t, \\
S_{Dij}(y|u_i) = \exp\{-u_i^\alpha \Lambda_0(y) \exp(\boldsymbol{\beta}_2' \mathbf{Z}_{2,ij})\}, & \Lambda_0(y) = \int_0^y \lambda_0(t)\mathrm{d}t.
\end{cases}
$$

The copula describes the intra-subject (individual-level) dependence between X_{ij} and D_{ij}. We mainly focus on modeling positive dependence between X_{ij} and D_{ij} using the Clayton or Gumbel copula[1]:

The Clayton copula

$$
C_\theta(v, w) = (v^{-\theta} + w^{-\theta} - 1)^{-1/\theta}, \quad \theta > 0,
$$

The Gumbel copula

$$
C_\theta(v, w) = \exp\left[-\{(-\log v)^{\theta+1} + (-\log w)^{\theta+1}\}^{\frac{1}{\theta+1}}\right], \quad \theta \geq 0.
$$

Copulas provide a simple way to compute measures of correlation between X_{ij} and D_{ij}. The most popular measure is Kendall's tau, though copulas can also provide other measures such as Spearman's rho.

Under the Clayton copula, Kendall's tau is $\tau_\theta = \theta/(\theta + 2)$.

Under the Gumbel copula, Kendall's tau is $\tau_\theta = \theta/(\theta + 1)$.

More details about copulas and Kendall's tau are referred to Sect. 2.6.

As in Burzykowski et al. (2001), one can use Kendall's tau as a measure of the individual-level dependence between two endpoints in meta-analysis.

---

[1] The Clayton copula can be extended to allow for negative dependence by setting $\theta < 0$. However, we do not consider such an extension since it produces a singular distribution (Nelsen 2006). The Gumbel copula cannot be defined for $\theta < 0$.

Under the independence copula $C_\theta(v, w) = vw$, Definition 2 reduces to the joint frailty model (Definition 1). Note that the Clayton and Gumbel copulas reduce to the independence copula by setting $\theta \to 0$.

One might also consider some copulas that allow negative dependence, such as the FGM copula

The Farlie–Gumbel–Morgenstern (FGM) copula:

$$C_\theta(v, w) = vw\{1 + \theta(1 - v)(1 - w)\}, \quad -1 \le \theta \le 1.$$

Under the FGM copula, Kendall's tau is $\tau_\theta = 2\theta/9$. However, the range of Kendall's tau is restricted from $\tau_{-1} = -2/9$ to $\tau_1 = 2/9$.

3.4 Penalized Likelihood with Splines

A likelihood function can be constructed given observed data $(T_{ij}, T_{ij}^*, \delta_{ij}, \delta_{ij}^*, \mathbf{Z}_{1,ij}, \mathbf{Z}_{2,ij})$ for $i = 1, 2, \ldots, G$ and $j = 1, 2, \ldots, N_i$. Define notations

$$R_{ij}(t) = R_0(t) \exp(\boldsymbol{\beta}_1' \mathbf{Z}_{1,ij}), \quad r_{ij}(t) = dR_{ij}(t)/dt = r_0(t) \exp(\boldsymbol{\beta}_1' \mathbf{Z}_{1,ij}),$$

$$\Lambda_{ij}(t) = \Lambda_0(t) \exp(\boldsymbol{\beta}_2' \mathbf{Z}_{2,ij}), \quad \lambda_{ij}(t) = d\Lambda_{ij}(t)/dt = \lambda_0(t) \exp(\boldsymbol{\beta}_2' \mathbf{Z}_{2,ij}).$$

Proposition 1 *Under the joint frailty-copula model, the log-likelihood is*

$$\ell = \sum_{i=1}^{G} \left[\sum_{j=1}^{N_i} \left\{ \delta_{ij} \log r_{ij}(T_{ij}) + \delta_{ij}^* \log \lambda_{ij}(T_{ij}^*) \right\} \right.$$

$$+ \log \int_0^\infty \left\{ u^{m_i + \alpha m_i^*} \prod_{j=1}^{N_i} \psi_\theta \left[uR_{ij}(T_{ij}), u^\alpha \Lambda_{ij}(T_{ij}^*) \right]^{\delta_{ij}} \psi_\theta^* \left[uR_{ij}(T_{ij}), u^\alpha \Lambda_{ij}(T_{ij}^*) \right]^{\delta_{ij}^*} \right.$$

$$\left. \left. \times \Theta_\theta \left[uR_{ij}(T_{ij}), u^\alpha \Lambda_{ij}(T_{ij}^*) \right]^{\delta_{ij}\delta_{ij}^*} D_\theta \left[uR_{ij}(T_{ij}), u^\alpha \Lambda_{ij}(T_{ij}^*) \right] \right\} f_\eta(u) du \right], \quad (3.3)$$

$$where, \ m_i = \sum_{j=1}^{N_i} \delta_{ij}, \ m_i^* = \sum_{j=1}^{N_i} \delta_{ij}^*, \ D_\theta[s,t] = C_\theta[\exp(-s), \exp(-t)],$$

$$\psi_\theta[s,t] = \frac{D_\theta^{[1,0]}[s,t]}{D_\theta[s,t]}, \ \psi_\theta^*[s,t] = \frac{D_\theta^{[0,1]}[s,t]}{D_\theta[s,t]}, \ \Theta_\theta[s,t] = \frac{D_\theta^{[1,1]}[s,t]D_\theta[s,t]}{D_\theta^{[1,0]}[s,t]D_\theta^{[0,1]}[s,t]},$$

$$D_\theta^{[1,0]}[s,t] = -\partial D_\theta[s,t]/\partial s, \ D_\theta^{[0,1]}[s,t] = -\partial D_\theta[s,t]/\partial t, \ and \ D_\theta^{[1,1]} = \partial^2 D_\theta[s,t]/\partial s \partial t.$$

Proof of Proposition 1: Let $\mathbf{T}_i = (T_{i1}, \ldots, T_{iN_i})$, $\mathbf{T}_i^* = (T_{i1}^*, \ldots, T_{iN_i}^*)$, $\boldsymbol{\delta}_i = (\delta_{i1}, \ldots, \delta_{iN_i})$, and $\boldsymbol{\delta}_i^* = (\delta_{i1}^*, \ldots, \delta_{iN_i}^*)$ be the data in the ith cluster. Given u_i, the likelihood for the ith study is

$$L(\mathbf{T}_i, \mathbf{T}_i^*, \boldsymbol{\delta}_i, \boldsymbol{\delta}_i^* | u_i) = \prod_{j=1}^{N_i} \Pr\Big(X_{ij} = T_{ij}, D_{ij} = T_{ij}^* | u_i\Big)^{\delta_{ij}\delta_{ij}^*} \Pr\Big(X_{ij} = T_{ij}, D_{ij} > T_{ij}^* | u_i\Big)^{\delta_{ij}(1-\delta_{ij}^*)}$$

$$\times \Pr\Big(X_{ij} > T_{ij}, D_{ij} = T_{ij}^* | u_i\Big)^{(1-\delta_{ij})\delta_{ij}^*} \Pr\Big(X_{ij} > T_{ij}, D_{ij} > T_{ij}^* | u_i\Big)^{(1-\delta_{ij})(1-\delta_{ij}^*)}$$

$$= \prod_{j=1}^{N_i} \left\{ u_i r_{ij}(T_{ij}) u_i^\alpha \lambda_{ij}\Big(T_{ij}^*\Big) D_\theta^{[1,1]}\Big[u_i R_{ij}(T_{ij}), u_i^\alpha \Lambda_{ij}\Big(T_{ij}^*\Big)\Big] \right\}^{\delta_{ij}\delta_{ij}^*}$$

$$\times \left\{ u_i r_{ij}(T_{ij}) D_\theta^{[1,0]}\Big[u_i R_{ij}(T_{ij}), u_i^\alpha \Lambda_{ij}\Big(T_{ij}^*\Big)\Big] \right\}^{\delta_{ij}-\delta_{ij}\delta_{ij}^*}$$

$$\times \left\{ u_i^\alpha \lambda_{ij}\Big(T_{ij}^*\Big) D_\theta^{[0,1]}\Big[u_i R_{ij}(T_{ij}), u_i^\alpha \Lambda_{ij}\Big(T_{ij}^*\Big)\Big] \right\}^{\delta_{ij}^*-\delta_{ij}\delta_{ij}^*}$$

$$\times \left\{ D_\theta\Big[u_i R_{ij}(T_{ij}), u_i^\alpha \Lambda_{ij}\Big(T_{ij}^*\Big)\Big] \right\}^{1-\delta_{ij}-\delta_{ij}^*+\delta_{ij}\delta_{ij}^*}$$

$$= \left\{ \prod_{j=1}^{N_i} r_{ij}(T_{ij})^{\delta_{ij}} \lambda_{ij}\Big(T_{ij}^*\Big)^{\delta_{ij}^*} \right\}$$

$$\times \left\{ u_i^{m_i+\alpha m_i^*} \prod_{j=1}^{N_i} \psi_\theta\Big[u_i R_{ij}(T_{ij}), u_i^\alpha \Lambda_{ij}\Big(T_{ij}^*\Big)\Big]^{\delta_{ij}} \psi_\theta^*\Big[u_i R_{ij}(T_{ij}), u_i^\alpha \Lambda_{ij}\Big(T_{ij}^*\Big)\Big]^{\delta_{ij}^*} \right.$$

$$\left. \times \Theta_\theta\Big[u_i R_{ij}(T_{ij}), u_i^\alpha \Lambda_{ij}(T_{ij}^*)\Big]^{\delta_{ij}\delta_{ij}^*} D_\theta\Big[u_i R_{ij}(T_{ij}), u_i^\alpha \Lambda_{ij}(T_{ij}^*)\Big] \right\}.$$

Integrating out the unobserved frailty, the likelihood for the ith study is

$$L(\mathbf{T}_i, \mathbf{T}_i^*, \boldsymbol{\delta}_i, \boldsymbol{\delta}_i^*) = \int_0^\infty L(\mathbf{T}_i, \mathbf{T}_i^*, \boldsymbol{\delta}_i, \boldsymbol{\delta}_i^* | u) f_\eta(u) du$$

$$= \prod_{j=1}^{N_i} r_{ij}(T_{ij})^{\delta_{ij}} \lambda_{ij}\Big(T_{ij}^*\Big)^{\delta_{ij}^*}$$

$$\times \int_0^\infty \left\{ u^{m_i+\alpha m_i^*} \prod_{j=1}^{N_i} \psi_\theta\Big[u R_{ij}(T_{ij}), u^\alpha \Lambda_{ij}\Big(T_{ij}^*\Big)\Big]^{\delta_{ij}} \psi_\theta^*\Big[u R_{ij}(T_{ij}), u^\alpha \Lambda_{ij}\Big(T_{ij}^*\Big)\Big]^{\delta_{ij}^*} \right.$$

$$\left. \times \Theta_\theta\Big[u R_{ij}(T_{ij}), u^\alpha \Lambda_{ij}\Big(T_{ij}^*\Big)\Big]^{\delta_{ij}\delta_{ij}^*} D_\theta\Big[u R_{ij}(T_{ij}), u^\alpha \Lambda_{ij}\Big(T_{ij}^*\Big)\Big] \right\} f_\eta(u) du.$$

Equation (3.3) follows by taking logarithm and summing up for $i = 1, 2, \ldots, G$ ∎.

The log-likelihood function in Eq. (3.3) has a simple form under the Clayton copula, one can easily obtain $D_\theta[s, t] = A_\theta(s, t)^{-1/\theta}$, $\psi_\theta[s, t] = \exp(\theta s)/A_\theta(s, t)$, $\psi_\theta^*[s, t] = \exp(\theta t)/A_\theta(s, t)$, and $\Theta_\theta[s, t] = 1 + \theta$, where $A_\theta(s, t) = \exp(\theta s) + \exp(\theta t) - 1$. By substituting these forms into Eq. (3.3), the log-likelihood is readily computable.

Following Rondeau et al. (2015), the forms of $r_0(\cdot)$ and $\lambda_0(\cdot)$ are modeled via the cubic *M-spline* (Ramsay 1988). The spline method aims to obtain smooth estimate for $r_0(\cdot)$ or $\lambda_0(\cdot)$ as a weighted sum of cubic polynomial functions, called basis functions. To define basis functions, one needs to determine knots that divide the range of observed event times (see Fig. 3.2 for example).

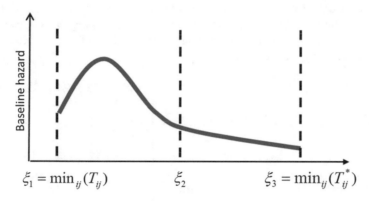

Fig. 3.2 A baseline hazard function expressed by the cubic M-spline. The knots are set by the smallest event time $\xi_1 = \min_{ij}(T_{ij})$, the largest follow-up time $\xi_3 = \min_{ij}(T_{ij}^*)$, and their intermediate value $\xi_2 = (\xi_1 + \xi_3)/2$

For instance, we define $r_0(t)$ and $\lambda_0(t)$ on $t \in [\xi_1, \xi_3]$, where $\xi_1 < \xi_2 < \xi_3$ are the knots. One may set the smallest event time $\xi_1 = \min_{ij}(T_{ij})$, the largest follow-up time $\xi_3 = \min_{ij}(T_{ij}^*)$, and $\xi_2 = (\xi_1 + \xi_3)/2$. We then obtain the five basis functions such that

$$r_0(t) = \sum_{\ell=1}^{5} g_\ell M_\ell(t) = \mathbf{g}'\mathbf{M}(t), \quad \lambda_0(t) = \sum_{\ell=1}^{5} h_\ell M_\ell(t) = \mathbf{h}'\mathbf{M}(t),$$

where $\mathbf{M}(t) = (M_1(t), \ldots, M_5(t))'$ are the M-spline basis functions and are cubic polynomial functions of t. The concrete formulas of the basis functions are given in Appendix A. Here, $\mathbf{g}' = (g_1, \ldots, g_5)$ and $\mathbf{h}' = (h_1, \ldots, h_5)$ are unknown positive parameters. The five-parameter model gives a good flexibility for real applications (Ramsay 1988) and is one of reasonable choices (Commenges and Jacqmin-Gadda 2015). Since the spline bases are easy to integrate, the baseline cumulative hazard functions are computed as

$$R_0(t) = \sum_{\ell=1}^{5} g_\ell I_\ell(t), \quad \Lambda_0(t) = \sum_{\ell=1}^{5} h_\ell I_\ell(t),$$

where $I_\ell(t)$ is the integration of $M_\ell(t)$, called the *I-spline* basis (Ramsay 1988).

The M-spline and I-spline bases are displayed in Fig. 2.1 of Chap. 2, and their expressions are given in Appendix A. The *joint.Cox* package offers functions *M.spline()* for computing $M_\ell(t)$ and *I.spline()* for $I_\ell(t)$.

With the spline-based model, we consider a penalized log-likelihood

$$\ell(\alpha, \eta, \theta, \boldsymbol{\beta}_1, \boldsymbol{\beta}_2, \mathbf{g}, \mathbf{h}) - \kappa_1 \int \ddot{r}_0(t)^2 \mathrm{d}t - \kappa_2 \int \ddot{\lambda}_0(t)^2 \mathrm{d}t, \tag{3.4}$$

where $\ddot{f}(t) = \mathrm{d}^2 f(t)/\mathrm{d}t^2$, and (κ_1, κ_2) are given nonnegative values. The parameters (κ_1, κ_2) are called smoothing parameters, which control the degrees of penalties on the roughness of the two baseline hazard functions. Under the five-parameter splines, it can be shown (Appendix A) that

$$\int \ddot{r}_0(t)^2 \mathrm{d}t = \mathbf{g}'\Omega\mathbf{g}, \int \ddot{\lambda}_0(t)^2 \mathrm{d}t = \mathbf{h}'\Omega\mathbf{h}, \Omega = \begin{bmatrix} 192 & -132 & 24 & 12 & 0 \\ -132 & 96 & -24 & -12 & 12 \\ 24 & -24 & 24 & -24 & 24 \\ 12 & -12 & -24 & 96 & -132 \\ 0 & 12 & 24 & -132 & 192 \end{bmatrix}.$$

Hence, the penalized log-likelihood is written as

$$\ell_{PL}(\alpha, \eta, \theta, \boldsymbol{\beta}_1, \boldsymbol{\beta}_2, \mathbf{g}, \mathbf{h}) = \ell(\alpha, \eta, \theta, \boldsymbol{\beta}_1, \boldsymbol{\beta}_2, \mathbf{g}, \mathbf{h}) - \kappa_1 \mathbf{g}'\Omega\mathbf{g} - \kappa_2 \mathbf{h}'\Omega\mathbf{h} \tag{3.5}$$

for a given pair of (κ_1, κ_2). We suggest choosing κ_1 and κ_2 by maximizing $\mathrm{LCV}_1(\kappa_1)$ and $\mathrm{LCV}_2(\kappa_2)$ that shall be defined in Sect. 3.7.

If $C_\theta(v, w) = vw$ is fitted (or if $\theta \approx 0$ is assumed in the Clayton copula), then the penalized log-likelihood in Eq. (3.5) is equivalent to that for the joint frailty model of Rondeau et al. (2015). See Exercise 6 for more details.

The standard error (SE) and confidence interval (CI) are calculated from the converged Hessian matrix defined as $\hat{H}_{PL} \equiv H_{PL}(\hat{\boldsymbol{\varphi}})$, where $H_{PL}(\boldsymbol{\varphi}) = \partial^2 \ell_{PL}(\boldsymbol{\varphi})/\partial \boldsymbol{\varphi}^2$ and $\hat{\boldsymbol{\varphi}} = (\hat{\eta}, \hat{\theta}, \hat{\boldsymbol{\beta}}_1, \hat{\boldsymbol{\beta}}_2, \hat{\mathbf{g}}, \hat{\mathbf{h}}) = \arg\max_{\boldsymbol{\varphi}} \ell_{PL}(\boldsymbol{\varphi})$. For instance, the 95% CI for β_1 is

$$\hat{\beta}_1 \pm 1.96 \times \mathrm{SE}(\hat{\beta}_1) = \hat{\beta}_1 \pm 1.96 \times \sqrt{(-\hat{H}_{PL}^{-1})_{\beta_1}}.$$

Similarly, the 95% CI for the baseline hazard function $r_0(x)$ is

$$\hat{r}_0(t) \pm 1.96 \times \mathrm{SE}\{\hat{r}_0(t)\} = \mathbf{M}'(t)\hat{\mathbf{g}} \pm 1.96 \times \sqrt{\mathbf{M}'(t)(-\hat{H}_{PL}^{-1})_{\mathbf{g}}\mathbf{M}(t)}.$$

One can use the *joint.Cox* R package (Emura 2019) for computing κ_1, κ_2, $\hat{\varphi}$, the SEs and 95%CIs.

3.5 Case Study: Ovarian Cancer Data

To demonstrate statistical methods introduced in this chapter, we analyze the subset of the ovarian cancer data of Ganzfried et al. (2013). Ganzfried et al. (2013) performed the IPD meta-analysis on their data to conclude that the gene expression of *CXCL12* is significantly associated with OS. In our analysis, we examine the effect of the *CXCL12* gene expression on time-to-relapse and OS using the joint frailty-copula model.

To this end, we chose the subset consisting of four studies that recorded the two endpoints as previously considered by Emura et al. (2017). Table 3.2 shows the subset containing 1003 ovarian cancer patients from the four studies ($N_1 = 110$, $N_2 = 58$, $N_3 = 278$, and $N_4 = 557$), which is available in the *joint.Cox* package. All patients are surgically treated and then followed up for cancer relapse until death or censoring. We regard TTP as time-to-relapse that is measured from the time of surgery. We consider the *CXCL12* gene expression as a covariate for TTP and OS.

Table 3.2 Data on ovarian cancer patients (Ganzfried et al. 2013; Emura et al. 2017)

Dataset[a]	Sample size	The number of observed events (event rates %)		
		Relapse ($\delta_{ij} = 1$)	Death ($\delta_{ij}^* = 1$)	Censoring ($\delta_{ij}^* = 0$)
GSE17260	$N_1 = 110$	76 (69%)	46 (42%)	64 (58%)
GSE30161	$N_2 = 58$	48 (83%)	36 (62%)	22 (38%)
GSE9891	$N_3 = 278$	185 (67%)	113 (41%)	165 (59%)
TCGA	$N_4 = 557$	266 (48%)	290 (52%)	267 (48%)
Total	$\sum_{i=1}^{4} N_i = 1003$	575 (57%)	485 (48%)	518 (52%)

Notes [a]Dataset is signified as GEO (Gene Expression Omnibus) accession number. Event rates (%) are the percentage of experiencing a particular event (Relapse, Death or Censoring) within a study

We fitted the joint frailty-copula model to the data by using R codes given in B1 of Appendix B. After running the codes, we obtained the plots for searching the optimal values of the smoothing parameters κ_1 and κ_2 (Fig. 3.3). One can see that $\kappa_1 = 2.76 \times 10^{16}$ and $\kappa_2 = 3.45 \times 10^{16}$ are chosen as the maximizers for $LCV_1(\kappa_1)$ and $LCV_2(\kappa_2)$, respectively.

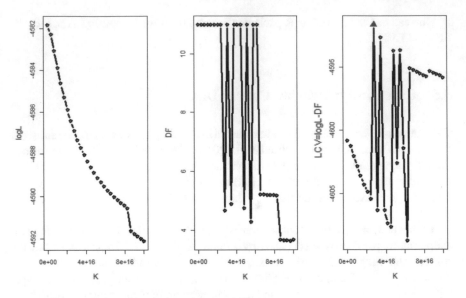

(1) The optimal value $\kappa_1 = 2.76 \times 10^{16}$ is shown in the rightmost panel.

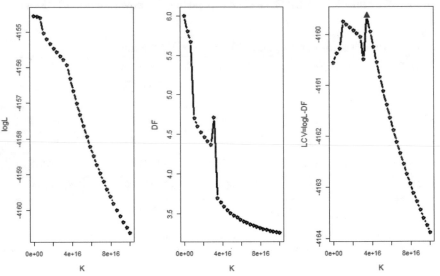

(2) The optimal value $\kappa_2 = 3.45 \times 10^{16}$ is shown in the rightmost panel.

Fig. 3.3 Plots for choosing the optimal values for κ_1 and κ_2. They are chosen by maximizing LCV = logL-DF, where logL is the log-likelihood and DF is the degrees of freedom

The outputs for the R codes are shown below

```
> res
$count
No.of samples  No.of events  No.of deaths  No.of censors
4          110          76           46           64
8           58          48           36           22
11         278         185          113          165
14         557         266          290          267


$beta1
   estimate           SE       Lower        Upper
0.19946579   0.03819308   0.12460735   0.27432422


$beta2
   estimate           SE       Lower        Upper
0.16550013   0.04371864   0.07981159   0.25118867


$eta
    estimate           SE        Lower         Upper
0.033423894   0.029324063   0.005987583   0.186578891


$theta
  estimate          SE       Lower        Upper
2.3468206   0.2500292   1.9045466   2.8917996


$tau
   estimate       tau_se       Lower        Upper
0.53989360   0.02646533   0.48777664   0.59115251


$LCV1
             K1            LCV1
2.758621e+16   -4.591564e+03


$LCV2
             K2            LCV2
3.448276e+16   -4.159635e+03


$g
[1] 9.065934e-01  1.711413e+00  6.733528e-06  3.947032e-02  2.790394e-07


$h
[1] 2.108053e-01  1.083808e+00  1.001098e+00  1.796956e-01  6.951190e-07


$g_var
                [,1]            [,2]            [,3]            [,4]            [,5]
[1,]  4.576008e-03  -3.369090e-03   1.552692e-07  -3.758267e-04   7.350478e-06
[2,] -3.369090e-03   2.656668e-02   2.655560e-08   6.202427e-04   1.600087e-05
[3,]  1.552692e-07   2.655560e-08  -2.475294e-07  -9.974754e-06  -1.157045e-08
[4,] -3.758267e-04   6.202427e-04  -9.974754e-06   5.863771e-02   8.841581e-06
[5,]  7.350478e-06   1.600087e-05  -1.157045e-08   8.841581e-06  -1.720272e-06


$h_var
                [,1]            [,2]            [,3]            [,4]            [,5]
[1,]  9.424816e-04  -1.368119e-03  -1.412362e-05  -7.147868e-04   4.058112e-10
[2,] -1.368119e-03   9.976173e-03  -1.180192e-02  -6.841087e-04  -4.529052e-10
[3,] -1.412362e-05  -1.180192e-02   5.718015e-02   2.243583e-03  -4.938438e-09
```

```
[4,] -7.147868e-04  -6.841087e-04   2.243583e-03   1.078262e-03  -2.439095e-10
[5,]  4.058112e-10  -4.529052e-10  -4.938438e-09  -2.439095e-10   7.476648e-15


$convergence
      MPL          DF          LCV      code  No.of.iterations  No.of.randomizations
-8604.09320  11.69913  -8610.04633  1.00000          98.00000              10.00000

$convergence.parameters
NULL
```

Now we interpret the above outputs.

In "$count" we see the sample size ("No. of samples" $= N_i$) and the number of events ("No. of events" $= m_i$, "No. of deaths" $= m_i^*$, "No. of censors" $= N_i - m_i^*$) in each study. The numbers in "$count" are the same as those available in Table 3.2. The numbers "4, 8, 11, 14" in the first column represent the study IDs, which do not have particular meaning[2].

From "$beta1" to "$tau", we see the estimate, the SE, and the 95%CI (lower and upper limits). The correspondences are "$beta1" $= \hat{\boldsymbol{\beta}}_1$, "$beta2" $= \hat{\boldsymbol{\beta}}_2$, "$eta"$= \hat{\eta}$, "$theta"$= \hat{\theta}$, and "$tau"$= \hat{\tau} = \hat{\theta}/(\hat{\theta} + 2)$. For instance, we had $\hat{\boldsymbol{\beta}}_1 = 0.199$ (95%CI: 0.125-0.274). These values are converted to RR $= \exp(\hat{\boldsymbol{\beta}}_1) = 1.22$ (95%CI: 1.13-1.32). We set $\alpha = 0$ in this analysis.

"$LCV1" and "$LCV2" show the results for the grid searches for maximizing $LCV_1(\kappa_1)$ and $LCV_2(\kappa_2)$, respectively. We see the maximizers $\kappa_1 = 2.76 \times 10^{16}$ and $\kappa_2 = 3.45 \times 10^{16}$ along with their maximized LCV values (see also Fig. 3.3).

"$g" and "$h" show the coefficients used in the splines, $\hat{\mathbf{g}}$ and $\hat{\mathbf{h}}$, respectively. The resultant baseline hazard functions are

$$\hat{r}_0(t) = 0.907 \times M_1(t) + 1.711 \times M_2(t) + 0.000 \times M_3(t) + 0.040 \times M_4(t) + 0.000 \times M_5(t),$$

$$\hat{\lambda}_0(t) = 0.211 \times M_1(t) + 1.084 \times M_2(t) + 1.001 \times M_3(t) + 0.180 \times M_4(t) + 0.000 \times M_5(t).$$

"$g_var" and "$h_var" are the covariance matrices of $\hat{\mathbf{g}}$ and $\hat{\mathbf{h}}$, which are equivalent to $(-\hat{H}_{PL}^{-1})_{\mathbf{g}}$ and $(-\hat{H}_{PL}^{-1})_{\mathbf{h}}$. They are used to compute the SEs and CIs of $\hat{r}_0(t)$ and $\hat{\lambda}_0(t)$.

"$convergence" shows several different aspects on likelihood maximization. "MPL" gives the maximized penalized log-likelihood in Eq. (3.5). "DF" gives the degrees of freedom that shall be defined in Sect. 3.7. The result "DF $= 11.69913$" implies that there are about 12 free parameters in the model. This number is smaller than the total number of parameters, $14 = 1 + 1 + 1 + 1 + 5 + 5$ (for $beta1, $beta2, $eta, $theta, $g and $h), owing to constrained (penalized) likelihood optimization. The value of "$LCV" represents the likelihood cross-validation (LCV) criterion, which is interpreted as the negative of AIC. A larger LCV value corresponds to a better model. Since the LCV value accounts for the number of parameters in the model, it can be used for variable selection. "Randomize_num $= 10$" implies that the default initial value did not converge, and so the package tried 10 different initial values

---

[2]These IDs are remnants of the study IDs previously used in an old version of the curatedOvarianData package. Since the IDs may be changed in the new versions, the ID numbers lost the meaning.

by adding random noises to the default initial values. The algorithm converged to the proper solution as indicated by "code $= 1$". This implies that the gradients of Eq. (3.5) are zero at the solution (see the help of the *nlm()* function in R).

Table 3.3 summarizes the outputs. The relative risk (RR) of *CXCL12* on OS is significantly greater than the null value (RR $= 1.18$, 95%CI: 1.08–1.29). The RR of *CXCL12* on time-to-relapse is even higher (RR $= 1.22$, 95%CI: 1.13–1.32) than that on OS. These RRs are relative to one standard deviation increase in the expression of *CXCL12*. Our result suggests that the expression of *CXCL12* is a potential biomarker predictive of cancer relapse in surgically treated ovarian cancer patients. The estimate of the copula parameter ($\hat{\theta} = 2.35$, 95%CI: 1.90–2.90) shows moderate amount of dependence between relapse and death ($\hat{\tau} = 0.54$, 95%CI: 0.38–0.70). This suggests that the cancer relapse may predict death in ovarian cancer patients.

Table 3.3 The joint analysis of time-to-relapse and OS using the meta-analytic data (four studies, 1003 patients) for ovarian cancer patients

	The Clayton copula	The independence copula
	Estimate (95% CI)	Estimate (95% CI)
RR^a for time-to-relapse: $\exp(\beta_1)$	1.22 (1.13–1.32)	1.24 (1.14–1.35)
RR^a for OS: $\exp(\beta_2)$	1.18 (1.08–1.29)	1.17 (1.07–1.29)
Heterogeneity: η	0.033 (0.006–0.187)	0.028 (0.004–0.180)
Copula parameter: θ	2.35 (1.90–2.90)	0.00 (fixed)
RR for death after relapse: $\theta + 1$	3.35 (2.90–3.90)	1.00 (fixed)
Kendall's tau: $\tau = \theta/(\theta + 2)$	0.54 (0.49–0.59)	–
Maximum penalized log-likelihood	−8604.09	−8744.02
Degrees of freedom	11.70	9.23
LCV^b	−8610.05	−8745.93

Notes [a]The RR (Relative Risk) of the *CXCL12* expression is examined (RR > 1 indicates that patients with high *CXCL12* expression have poor survival outcomes)
[b]The LCV (likelihood cross-validation) assesses model adequacy (larger LCV corresponds to better model)

Table 3.3 also includes the results under the independence copula (i.e., with a fixed copula parameter, $\theta \approx 0$). Due to the failure to account for residual dependence between time-to-relapse and OS, the LCV value under the independence model is smaller than that under the Clayton copula. Nevertheless, the estimates of RR are fairly comparable to those under the Clayton copula. This implies the robustness for marginal inference under copula misspecification. The simulation studies of Emura et al. (2017) also demonstrated some robustness for marginal inference against copula misspecification.

Once the fitted parameter values are obtained, one can display the estimated baseline hazard functions using the R codes given in B1 of Appendix B. Figure 3.4 plots the estimated baseline hazard functions $\hat{r}_0(t)$ and $\hat{\lambda}_0(t)$ and their 95% CIs. The baseline hazard rate for relapse ($\hat{r}_0(t)$) is high on early stage and gradually

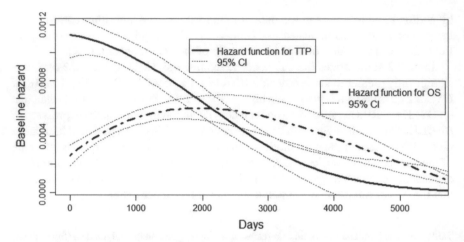

Fig. 3.4 Estimated baseline hazard functions for time-to-relapse (TTP) and overall survival (OS) in ovarian cancer patients

decreases as time passes. On the other hand, the hazard rate for death $(\hat{\lambda}_0(t))$ is initially low and reaches a peak at around 2000 days. Hereafter, the hazard rate of death is consistently higher than that of relapse. From these plots, one may suggest physicians monitoring patients carefully for cancer relapse before 2000 days, and after 2000 days, shifting more attention to other life-threatening symptoms. The possibility of the joint assessments of the two hazard functions is one of the crucial advantages of adopting splines for estimating baseline hazard functions.

3.6 Technical Note 1: Numerical Maximization

This section explains how the penalized log-likelihood in Eq. (3.5) is maximized in the *joint.Cox* R package.

To avoid constraints on parameters (e.g., $\theta > 0$), we consider log-transformed parameters $\tilde{\eta} = \log(\eta)$, $\tilde{\theta} = \log(\theta)$, $\tilde{\mathbf{g}} = \log(\mathbf{g})$ and $\tilde{\mathbf{h}} = \log(\mathbf{h})$. Given a value of α, one can write

$$\ell_{PL}(\eta, \theta, \boldsymbol{\beta}_1, \boldsymbol{\beta}_2, \mathbf{g}, \mathbf{h}) = \ell_{PL}(\exp(\tilde{\eta}), \exp(\tilde{\theta}), \boldsymbol{\beta}_1, \boldsymbol{\beta}_2, \exp(\tilde{\mathbf{g}}), \exp(\tilde{\mathbf{h}})) = \tilde{\ell}_{PL}(\tilde{\eta}, \tilde{\theta}, \boldsymbol{\beta}_1, \boldsymbol{\beta}_2, \tilde{\mathbf{g}}, \tilde{\mathbf{h}}).$$

A minimization function *nlm()* is applied to $-\tilde{\ell}_{PL}$ with the initial values $(\tilde{\eta}, \tilde{\theta}, \boldsymbol{\beta}_1, \boldsymbol{\beta}_2, \tilde{\mathbf{g}}, \tilde{\mathbf{h}}) = \mathbf{0}$. The initial values are equivalent to $\eta = \theta = 1$, $\boldsymbol{\beta}_1 = \boldsymbol{\beta}_2 = \mathbf{0}$, and $\mathbf{g} = \mathbf{h} = (1, 1, 1, 1, 1)'$. The converged Hessian matrix is defined as $\hat{H}_{PL} \equiv H_{PL}(\hat{\boldsymbol{\varphi}})$, where $H_{PL}(\boldsymbol{\varphi}) = \partial^2 \ell_{PL}(\boldsymbol{\varphi})/\partial \boldsymbol{\varphi}^2$ and $\hat{\boldsymbol{\varphi}} = (\hat{\eta}, \hat{\theta}, \hat{\boldsymbol{\beta}}_1, \hat{\boldsymbol{\beta}}_2, \hat{\mathbf{g}}, \hat{\mathbf{h}}) = \arg\max_{\boldsymbol{\varphi}} \ell_{PL}(\boldsymbol{\varphi})$. We obtain $\hat{H}_{PL}$ by multiplying an appropriate *transformation factor* to the output of *nlm(,hessian = TRUE)*. Note that $\hat{H}_{PL}$ is useful for calculating the SEs and LCV. If either *nlm()* does not converge or $\hat{H}_{PL}$ is not negative definite, the package tries different initial values by adding uniform random noises between -1 and 1 to $(\tilde{\eta}, \tilde{\theta}, \boldsymbol{\beta}_1, \boldsymbol{\beta}_2, \tilde{\mathbf{g}}, \tilde{\mathbf{h}}) = \mathbf{0}$, and then reapply *nlm()*. This idea of random initial values has been adopted in many different contexts (e.g., Hu and Emura 2015; Emura and Pan 2017). To calculate the integrals in Eq. (3.3), a numerical integration function *integrate()* is applied to the range $0 \leq u \leq 10$. To determine the value of α, one may use a profile likelihood, or try a few plausible values of α (e.g., $\alpha = 0$ or $\alpha = 1$).

3.7 Technical Note 2: LCV and Choice of κ_1 and κ_2

We define a likelihood cross-validation (LCV) criterion

$$\text{LCV} = \hat{\ell} - \text{tr}\{\hat{H}_{PL}^{-1}\hat{H}\},$$

where $\hat{\ell}$ is the log-likelihood value in Eq. (3.3) evaluated at $\hat{\boldsymbol{\varphi}}$, $\hat{H}_{PL}$ is the converged Hessian matrix of the penalized log-likelihood, and $\hat{H}$ is the converged Hessian matrix of the un-penalized log-likelihood. Specifically, $\hat{\ell} = \ell(\hat{\boldsymbol{\varphi}})$, $\hat{H}_{PL} = H_{PL}(\hat{\boldsymbol{\varphi}})$, and $\hat{H} = H(\hat{\boldsymbol{\varphi}})$, where $H(\boldsymbol{\varphi}) = \partial^2 \ell(\boldsymbol{\varphi})/\partial\boldsymbol{\varphi}^2$. The term $\text{tr}\{\hat{H}_{PL}^{-1}\hat{H}\}$ is the degrees of freedom, a decreasing function with increasing κ_1 and κ_2. The LCV is a criterion capable of choosing the best values of κ_1 and κ_2, as well as selecting the best subset of covariates. The LCV plays a similar role as the AIC for model selection. However, the calculation of the LCV requires high computational cost.

To alleviate the computational cost, we consider an approximation to the LCV in the following way. Under the working assumptions for the absence of heterogeneity and for the independence copula, the log-likelihood in Eq. (3.3) is

$$\ell(\boldsymbol{\beta}_1, \boldsymbol{\beta}_2, \mathbf{g}, \mathbf{h}) = \ell_1(\boldsymbol{\beta}_1, \mathbf{g}) + \ell_2(\boldsymbol{\beta}_2, \mathbf{h}),$$

where

$$\ell_1(\boldsymbol{\beta}_1, \mathbf{g}) = \sum_{i=1}^{G}\sum_{j=1}^{N_i} \{\delta_{ij} \log r_{ij}(T_{ij}) - R_{ij}(T_{ij})\}, \quad \ell_2(\boldsymbol{\beta}_2, \mathbf{h}) = \sum_{i=1}^{G}\sum_{j=1}^{N_i} \{\delta_{ij}^* \log \lambda_{ij}(T_{ij}^*) - \Lambda_{ij}(T_{ij}^*)\},$$

This suggests choosing κ_1 and κ_2 based on two separate Cox models. As detailed in Sect. 2.4.1, one can obtain penalized likelihood estimates $(\hat{\boldsymbol{\beta}}_1^{\text{PL}}, \hat{\mathbf{g}})$ and $(\hat{\boldsymbol{\beta}}_2^{\text{PL}}, \hat{\mathbf{h}})$ given κ_1 and κ_2 by using *splineCox.reg()*. Then, we define two LCVs

$$\text{LCV}_1 = \hat{\ell}_1 - \text{tr}\{\hat{H}_{PL1}^{-1}\hat{H}_1\}, \quad LCV_2 = \hat{\ell}_2 - \text{tr}\{\hat{H}_{PL2}^{-1}\hat{H}_2\},$$

where $\hat{\ell}_1$ and $\hat{\ell}_2$ are the log-likelihood values evaluated at their penalized likelihood estimates, and $\hat{H}_{PL1}$ and $\hat{H}_{PL2}$ are the converged Hessian matrices for the penalized likelihood estimations, $\hat{H}_1$ and $\hat{H}_2$ are the converged Hessian matrices for the log-likelihoods such that

$$\hat{H}_1 = \hat{H}_{PL1} + 2\kappa_1 \begin{bmatrix} O_{p_1 \times p_1} & O_{p_1 \times 5} \\ O_{5 \times p_1} & \Omega \end{bmatrix}, \quad \hat{H}_2 = \hat{H}_{PL2} + 2\kappa_2 \begin{bmatrix} O_{p_2 \times p_2} & O_{p_2 \times 5} \\ O_{5 \times p_2} & \Omega \end{bmatrix},$$

where O is a zero matrix. We then expect that the following approximation holds:

$$\text{LCV} \approx \text{LCV}_1 + \text{LCV}_2.$$

Consequently, maximizing LCV is roughly equal to maximizing LCV_1 for κ_1 and LCV_2 for κ_2, separately.

The *joint.Cox* package provides the plots of LCV_1 and LCV_2 on a given grid along with the optimized values for κ_1 and κ_2. When looking at the outputs, following properties must be checked: (i) $\hat{\ell}_1$ and $\hat{\ell}_2$ are smoothly decreasing in κ_1 and κ_2, respectively, (ii) the degrees of freedom $\text{tr}\{\hat{H}_{PL1}^{-1}\hat{H}_1\}$ decreases from p_1+5 to p_1+2; the degrees of freedom $\text{tr}\{\hat{H}_{PL2}^{-1}\hat{H}_2\}$ decreases from p_2+5 to p_2+2. If these two properties are not met, the grid is inappropriate. The degrees of freedoms can occasionally be quite big if the Hessian matrix is singular. The values of κ_1 and κ_2 producing such results are ignored.

Given the chosen values for κ_1 or κ_2, we fit the joint frailty-copula model and calculate $LCV = \hat{\ell} - \text{tr}\{\hat{H}_{PL}^{-1}\hat{H}\}$. The LCV represents the trade-off between goodness-of-fit ($\hat{\ell}$) and the degrees of freedom ($\text{tr}\{\hat{H}_{PL}^{-1}\hat{H}\}$). Hence, the LCV is similar to the AIC. Consequently, the LCV can be used for covariate selection. That is, the best subset of covariates is the one that minimizes the LCV. While one has LCV $\approx$ $\text{LCV}_1 + \text{LCV}_2$, the values of LCV_1 and LCV_2 are used in order only to choose κ_1 and κ_2.

3.8 Exercises

1. Consider the joint frailty model with $\alpha = 1$, that is,

    $$\Pr(X_{ij} > x, D_{ij} > y|u_i) = \exp\left[-u_i\{R_{ij}(x) + \Lambda_{ij}(y)\}\right].$$

    Show $\Pr(X_{ij} > x, D_{ij} > y) = [1 + \eta\{R_{ij}(x) + \Lambda_{ij}(y)\}]^{-1/\eta}$ under the gamma frailty model.

2. Consider the joint frailty-copula model in Eq. (3.2) with $\alpha = 1$ and the Gumbel copula,

    $$\Pr(X_{ij} > x, D_{ij} > y|u_i) = \exp\left[-u_i\{R_{ij}(x)^{\theta+1} + \Lambda_{ij}(y)^{\theta+1}\}^{1/(1+\theta)}\right].$$

    Derive the expression of $\Pr(X_{ij} > x, D_{ij} > y)$.

3. Consider the joint frailty-copula model in Eq. (3.2) with $\alpha = 1$ and the Clayton copula,

    $$\Pr(X_{ij} > x, D_{ij} > y|u_i) = \left[\exp\{\theta u_i R_{ij}(x)\} + \exp\{\theta u_i \Lambda_{ij}(y)\} - 1\right]^{-1/\theta}.$$

(1) Under $\eta = 1$, derive the expression of $\Pr(X_{ij} > x, D_{ij} > y)$ by using
$$H_\theta(a, b) = \int_0^1 \left(t^{-a\theta} + t^{-b\theta} - 1\right)^{-1/\theta} dt.$$

(2) Derive the expression of $\Pr(X_{ij} > x, D_{ij} > y)$ by using some function $H_{\eta,\theta}(a, b)$.

4. Consider the joint frailty-copula model in Eq. (3.2) with $\alpha = 1$ and the Pareto baseline hazard functions,

$$r_0(x) = \gamma_1/x, \quad \gamma_1 > 0, \quad x \geq \xi_1 > 0,$$
$$\lambda_0(y) = \gamma_2/y, \quad \gamma_2 > 0, \quad y \geq \xi_2 > 0.$$

Derive the expression of $\Pr(X_{ij} > x, D_{ij} > y | u_i)$ under the Clayton and Gumbel copulas.

5. Show the relationship between $\Theta_\theta[s, t]$ and $R_\theta[u, v]$ that is defined in Sect. 2.6.

6. Under the independence copula $C_\theta(v, w) = vw$, show that Eq. (3.3) reduces to the log-likelihood of Rondeau et al. (2015) as follows:

$$\ell(\alpha, \eta, \beta_1, \beta_2, r_0, \lambda_0) = \sum_{i=1}^{G} \left[\sum_{j=1}^{N_i} \left\{ \delta_{ij} \log r_{ij}(T_{ij}) + \delta_{ij}^* \log \lambda_{ij}(T_{ij}^*) \right\} \right.$$
$$\left. + \log \int_0^\infty \left\{ u^{m_i + \alpha m_i^*} \exp\left(-u \sum_{j=1}^{N_i} R_{ij}(T_{ij}) - u^\alpha \sum_{j=1}^{N_i} \Lambda_{ij}(T_{ij}^*) \right) \right\} f_\eta(u) du \right].$$

Simplify the above expression when $\alpha = 0$ and $\alpha = 1$, respectively.

7. Derive $D_\theta[s, t]$, $\psi_\theta[s, t]$, $\psi_\theta^*[s, t]$, and $\Theta_\theta[s, t]$ under the Gumbel copula.

8. Do the above exercise under the Farlie–Gumbel–Morgenstern (FGM) copula.

9. When performing numerical integrations in Eq. (3.3), we used the truncated range $0 \leq u \leq 10$ rather than $0 \leq u < \infty$. This avoids some instability occurring for $u > 10$.

(1) Draw a figure to show the gamma density for $0 \leq u \leq 10$ under several parameter values. Compare your figure with the figure given by Aalen (1994).

(2) Conduct a numerical experiment to demonstrate if the range $0 \leq u \leq 10$ is enough to evaluate the integrations in the log-likelihood.

10. Let $\ell(\varphi)$ be a function of φ, and $\tilde{\ell}(\tilde{\varphi})$ be defined as $\tilde{\ell}(\tilde{\varphi}) = \ell(e^{\tilde{\varphi}})$. Also, let $\tilde{S}(\tilde{\varphi}) = \partial \tilde{\ell}(\tilde{\varphi})/\partial \tilde{\varphi}$ and $\tilde{H}(\tilde{\varphi}) = \partial^2 \tilde{\ell}(\tilde{\varphi})/\partial \tilde{\varphi}^2$. Write $S(\tilde{\varphi}) = \partial \ell(\tilde{\varphi})/\partial \tilde{\varphi}$ and $H(\tilde{\varphi}) = \partial^2(\tilde{\varphi})/\partial \tilde{\varphi}^2$ in terms of $\tilde{S}(\cdot)$ and $\tilde{H}(\cdot)$. Write down "a transformation factor" mentioned in Sect. 3.6.

References

Aalen OO (1994) Effects of frailty in survival analysis. Stat Methods Med Res 3(3):227–243

Burzykowski T, Molenberghs G, Buyse M, Geys H, Renard D (2001) Validation of surrogate end points in multiple randomized clinical trials with failure time end points. Appl Stat 50(4):405–422

Burzykowski T, Molenberghs G, Buyse M (eds) (2005) The evaluation of surrogate endpoints. Springer, New York

Commenges D, Jacqmin-Gadda H (2015) Dynamical biostatistical models. CRC Press, London

Emura T, Nakatochi M, Murotani K, Rondeau V (2017) A joint frailty-copula model between tumour progression and death for meta-analysis. Stat Methods Med Res 26(6):2649–2666

Emura T (2019). joint.Cox: joint frailty-copula models for tumour progression and death in meta-analysis, CRAN

Emura T, Pan CH (2017) Parametric likelihood inference and goodness-of-fit for dependently left-truncated data, a copula-based approach, Stat Pap https://doi.org/10.1007/s00362-017-0947-z

Fine JP, Jiang H, Chappell R (2001) On semi-competing risks data. Biometrika 88:907–920

Ganzfried BF, Riester M, Haibe-Kains B et al (2013) Curated ovarian data: clinically annotated data for the ovarian cancer transcriptome, Database; Article ID bat013: https://doi.org/10.1093/database/bat013

Haneuse S, Lee KH (2016) Semi-competing risks data analysis, accounting for death as a competing risk when the outcome of interest is nonterminal. Circ Cardiovasc Qual Outcomes 9:322–331

Hu YH, Emura T (2015) Maximum likelihood estimation for a special exponential family under random double-truncation. Computation Stat 30(4):1199–1229

Nelsen RB (2006) An introduction to copulas, 2nd edn. Springer, New York

Peng M, Xiang L, Wang S (2018) Semiparametric regression analysis of clustered survival data with semi-competing risks. Comput Stat Data Anal 124:53–70

Ramsay J (1988) Monotone regression spline in action. Statis Sci 3:425–461

Rondeau V, Pignon JP, Michiels S (2015) A joint model for dependence between clustered times to tumour progression and deaths: a meta-analysis of chemotherapy in head and neck cancer. Stat Methods Med Res 24(6):711–729

Rotolo F, Paoletti X, Michiels S (2018) surrosurv: an R package for the evaluation of failure time surrogate endpoints in individual patient data meta-analyses of randomized clinical trials. Comput Methods Programs Biomed 155:189–198

Chapter 4
High-Dimensional Covariates in the Joint Frailty-Copula Model

Abstract The concerns for over-fitting, high computational cost, and large estimation error arise when the number of covariates is large in a model. We introduce a simple and effective strategy to handle high-dimensional covariates based on Tukey's *compound covariate* method. We then demonstrate how the compound covariate method is applied to the joint frailty-copula model, and how patient-level survival is predicted. Using simulations, we compare the compound covariate method with ridge- and Lasso-based methods in a prediction setting. We analyze the ovarian cancer data for illustration.

Keywords Compound covariate · Cox regression · Feature selection · Gene expression · Univariate selection · Lasso · Meta-analysis · Ridge regression · Survival prediction

4.1 Introduction

In the presence of high-dimensional covariates, the traditional Cox regression analysis (Cox 1972) fails to provide a satisfactory result. Many techniques to overcome the problem for the traditional Cox model are now available (Witten and Tibshirani 2010). In particular, shrinkage techniques, such as ridge regression and Lasso, are commonly used to incorporate high-dimensional covariates into the Cox model (Bøvelstad et al. 2007).

These techniques developed for the Cox model employ the partial likelihood function, and hence they are not directly applicable to the joint frailty-copula model for correlated endpoints (Emura et al. 2017; Chap. 3). What we present in this chapter is the idea of *compound covariate* as advocated by Tukey (1993), a simple and effective strategy to handle high-dimensional covariates using the univariate Cox model.

Unlike shrinkage methods, the compound covariate method applies a univariate feature selection method using multiple tests. This method involves computation of the significance levels of features (in terms of P-value) and is suitable toward the objective of achieving biological insights, where screening of prognostic features

© The Author(s), under exclusive license to Springer Nature Singapore Pte Ltd. 2019   59
T. Emura et al., *Survival Analysis with Correlated Endpoints*,
JSS Research Series in Statistics, https://doi.org/10.1007/978-981-13-3516-7_4

exhaustively may be a relevant task, even if some selected features are highly correlated. In some shrinkage-based methods, such as Lasso, a feature subset may be
identified, taking account of the correlations among features. One has to recognize
that such a subset is one, haphazardly selected (due to random errors) from many
"solutions" of predictor with comparable predictive capability in high-dimensional
situations (Schumacher et al. 2012).

This chapter is organized as follows. Sections 4.2 and 4.3 review Tukey's compound covariate method. Section 4.4 introduces the data structure. Section 4.5 demonstrates how the compound covariate method is applied to the joint frailty-copula
model. Section 4.6 introduces the ridge regression and Lasso methods. Section 4.7
constructs the patient-level survival function for prediction. Section 4.8 conducts
simulation studies and Sect. 4.9 analyzes real data. Section 4.10 concludes with
discussions.

4.2   Tukey's Compound Covariate

The term *compound covariate* is first employed by Tukey (1993) who is also known
as the founder of the *jackknife method* and *exploratory data analysis*. According to
Tukey, compound covariate refers to a composite score calculated as a weighted sum
of individual covariates, where the weight assigned for each covariate is determined
by its univariate association with the outcome of interest. The compound covariate
method is a general method applicable to many different settings, including linear
regression, binary classification, logistic regression, and Cox regression.

We introduce Tukey's compound covariate as a tool for predicting survival.
Consider a future patient with a covariate vector $(Z_1, \ldots, Z_q)$. To predict clinical outcomes of the patient, one can consider a compound covariate, defined
as $w_1 Z_1 + \cdots + w_q Z_q$, where $(w_1, \ldots, w_q)$ is a vector of weights. In the compound covariate, the weight w_j is computed by fitting survival data to univariate
models, e.g., the partial likelihood estimate $w_j = \hat{\beta}_j$ under the univariate Cox
model $h_j(t|Z_j) = h_{0j}(t) \exp(\beta_j Z_j)$ for $j = 1, \ldots, p$. Some researchers apply
$w_j = \hat{\beta}_j / SE(\hat{\beta}_j)$ (Wang et al. 2005) or the Z-value of the score tests for w_j (Matsui
2006; Emura et al. 2019). In all cases, the compound covariate predictor is an
ensemble of univariate analyses, which does not employ a multivariate analysis.

If $w_j = \hat{\beta}_j$ is employed, high (low) value of the compound covariate is associated
with poor (good) prognosis for survival. This prediction method is called *compound
covariate prediction*. For instance, Chen et al. (2007) employed the weights $w_j = \hat{\beta}_j$
attached to the $q = 16$ gene expressions to construct a compound covariate

$$
\begin{aligned}
CC = &(-1.09 \times \text{ANXA5}) + (1.32 \times \text{DLG2}) + (0.55 \times \text{ZNF264}) + (0.75 \times \text{DUSP6}) \\
&+ (0.59 \times \text{CPEB4}) + (-0.84 \times \text{LCK}) + (-0.58 \times \text{STAT1}) + (0.65 \times \text{RNF4}) \\
&+ (0.52 \times \text{IRF4}) + (0.58 \times \text{STAT2}) + (0.51 \times \text{HGF}) + (0.55 \times \text{ERBB3}) \\
&+ (0.47 \times \text{NF1}) + (-0.77 \times \text{FRAP1}) + (0.92 \times \text{MMD}) + (0.52 \times \text{HMMR}),
\end{aligned}
$$

where the covariates are expressed in the gene symbols. This compound covariate predicts survival prognosis for lung cancer patients.

Compound covariate prediction has been shown to be useful in medical studies with gene expressions as a simple and powerful tool for survival prediction (Beer et al. 2002; Wang et al. 2005; Matsui 2006; Chen et al. 2007; Matsui et al. 2012; Emura et al. 2012, 2018, 2019; Zhao et al. 2014). The compound covariate method has the competitive performance over more sophisticated multivariate techniques, such as ridge and Lasso methods; see numerical studies of Emura et al. (2012, 2018, 2019) and Zhao et al. (2014).

4.3 Univariate Feature Selection

Since the compound covariate method utilizes univariate regression, it is closely related to *univariate feature selection* (Witten and Tibshirani 2010; Emura et al. 2019).

Suppose we wish to select a small fraction of genes from a large number of genes. Let p be the number of all available genes, where p can be large, such as $p \approx 5,000$. *Univariate feature selection* proceeds as follows: For each $j = 1, \ldots, p$, the null hypothesis $H_0 : \beta_j = 0$ is examined by the Wald test (or score test) under the univariate Cox model treating the j-th gene as a covariate. The parameter β_j represents the univariate association between survival and the gene, where all other genes are ignored. Then, one picks out a subset of genes that have low P-values from the tests. The top q $(< p)$ genes with lowest P-values are then selected.

Simon (2003) recommended the P-value threshold of 0.001 in microarrays analyses. This is more stringent than the traditional 0.01 or 0.05 criterion, but less stringent than the genome-wide significance 5×10^{-8}. The P-value < 0.001 condition is designed to allow some, but not too many false positives. For $p = 5000$, one would have $5000 \times 0.001 = 5$ falsely identified genes. See also Matsui et al. (2012) and Emura et al. (2018) who used the P-value threshold of 0.001 in analysis of survival data. For simplicity, we shall adopt the P-value threshold of 0.001.[1]

After selecting the q genes having P-values lower than the threshold, they are used to compute a compound covariate predictor $\sum_j \hat{\beta}_j Z_j$.

Remarkably, the prediction performance of the compound covariate predictor is robust against a small change in the P-value threshold. First, a small change of the P-value may not change the selected genes at all. This reason shall be illustrated by a simulation. Second, even if the selected genes are changed, majority of the genes with lower P-values are still kept in the predictor. This property is due to the *additive* property of the compound covariate predictor, without incorporating the correlations among genes. Many shrinkage methods, in particular, the Lasso, do not possess

---

[1]Obviously, the adequacy of 0.001 depends on many factors, such as the total number of genes and sample sizes. If one uses the *compound.Cox* R package, one can obtain a data-driven P-value threshold through a cross-validation (Emura et al. 2019).

this property since a small change in the shrinkage parameter can alter the whole structure of the predictor. The gain in predictive accuracy by ignoring correlations among high-dimensional gene expressions has been known in linear discriminant analysis (Dudoit et al. 2002; Bickel and Levina 2004).

An important caution is that one should not refit the multivariate Cox model after univariate selection (e.g., Lossos et al. 2004). If one refits the multivariate Cox model, some regression coefficients of the selected genes become nonsignificant, especially those among correlated genes. While many biomedical researchers prefer a multivariate prognostic model to avoid correlated genes in the model, the refitted model may lose predictive power (Bøvelstad et al. 2007; van Wieringen et al. 2009) and the additive property of the compound covariate predictor. Compound covariate prediction should be made by an aggregation of the univariate models without going through any multivariate model.

4.4 Meta-Analytic Data with High-Dimensional Covariates

The compound covariate method adapts to different types of analyses. Here, we consider an individual-patient data (IPD) meta-analysis of semi-competing risks data (Chap. 3). The semi-competing risks mean that a terminal event (death) censors a nonterminal event (tumour progression), but not vice versa. We also consider high-dimensional covariates that may be associated with both the terminal and nonterminal events.

Meta-analytic data consist of G independent studies with the i-th study containing N_i patients. For $i = 1, 2, \ldots, G$ and $j = 1, 2, \ldots, N_i$, let

- X_{ij}: time-to-tumour progression (TTP),
- D_{ij}: overall survival (OS), or equivalently, time-to-death,
- C_{ij}: independent and non-informative censoring time.

As explained in Chap. 3, what we actually observe are the semi-competing risks data $(T_{ij}, T_{ij}^*, \delta_{ij}, \delta_{ij}^*, \mathbf{Z}_{1,ij}, \mathbf{Z}_{2,ij}, \mathbf{U}_{ij})$ for $i = 1, 2, \ldots, G$ and $j = 1, 2, \ldots, N_i$, where

- $T_{ij} = \min(X_{ij}, D_{ij}, C_{ij})$: first-occurring event time,
- $\delta_{ij} = \mathbf{I}(T_{ij} = X_{ij})$: status of tumour progression (no progression $= 0$; progression $= 1$), where $\mathbf{I}(\cdot)$ is the indicator function,
- $T_{ij}^* = \min(D_{ij}, C_{ij})$: censored terminal event time,
- $\delta_{ij}^* = \mathbf{I}(T_{ij}^* = D_{ij})$: status for death (alive $= 0$; dead $= 1$),
- $\mathbf{Z}_{1,ij}$: p_1-dimensional clinical covariates associated with TTP,
- $\mathbf{Z}_{2,ij}$: p_2-dimensional clinical covariates associated with OS,
- $\mathbf{U}_{ij} = (U_{ij,1}, \ldots, U_{ij,p})$: p-dimensional gene expressions that are standardized to have mean $= 0$ and SD $= 1$ across the entire patients (or across patients within each study).

We assume that the numbers p_1 and p_2 are small and the number p is large.

Table 4.1 shows an example of the data used in Emura et al. (2018) consisting of 912 ovarian cancer patients from four independent studies. There are 11,756 gene expressions that are commonly available across the four studies. It is of our interest to examine how the gene expressions can be incorporated into a joint model for the terminal event (death) and nonterminal event (relapse).

Table 4.1 Meta-analytic data from four independent studies of ovarian cancer patients

Dataset[a]	Median follow-up (days)	Sample size	The number of observed events (event rates)			The number of genes
			Relapse $\left(\delta_{ij} = 1\right)$	Death $\left(\delta_{ij}^* = 1\right)$	Censoring $\left(\delta_{ij}^* = 0\right)$	
GSE17260	1410	$N_1 = 84$	59 (70%)	38 (45%)	46 (55%)	18,548
GSE30161	2513	$N_2 = 58$	48 (83%)	36 (62%)	22 (38%)	18,524
GSE9891	1140	$N_3 = 260$	185 (71%)	113 (43%)	147 (57%)	18,524
TCGA	1721	$N_4 = 510$	252 (49%)	278 (55%)	232 (45%)	12,211
Total		$\sum_{i=1}^{4} N_i = 912$	544 (60%)	465 (51%)	447 (49%)	Common = 11,756

Note The data are extracted from the *curatedOvarianData* package of Ganzfried et al. (2013)
[a]Dataset is signified as the GEO accession number which can be used to search the public genomics data in the GEO (Gene Expression Omnibus) repository. Extracted studies are the subset having documented values of "days-to-tumour-recurrence", "days-to-death", "recurrence status", and "vital status" for all patients. The median follow-up time is calculated from the Kaplan–Meier survival curve for time-to-censoring for each study. The event rates are calculated separately for each study. However, our data extraction yielded a slightly reduced list of patients compared to Table 3.2. The reason may be due to the update of "patientselection.config" file (from older version 1.0.3 to the version 1.8.0) in the package to remove some duplicate samples (Waldron et al. 2014)

4.5 The Joint Model with Compound Covariates

This section considers a method for fitting the data to the joint frailty-copula model for TTP and OS by screening the high-dimensional gene expressions $\mathbf{U}_{ij} = (U_{ij,1}, \ldots, U_{ij,p})$.

In the initial step, we select $q_1(< p)$ genes univariately associated with TTP based on the P-value < 0.001 criterion. More precisely, the data $\{(T_{ij}, \delta_{ij}, U_{ij,k}); i = 1, \ldots, G, j = 1, \ldots, N_i\}$ are fitted to the univariate Cox model for TTP, say $r_{ij,k}(t) = r_{0,k}(t) \exp(b_k U_{ij,k})$, and the P-value of testing the null hypothesis $H_0 : b_k = 0$ is evaluated on the k-th gene ($k = 1, \ldots, p$). Similarly, we select $q_2(< p)$ genes univariately associated with OS based on the data $\{(T_{ij}^*, \delta_{ij}^*, U_{ij,k}); i = 1, \ldots, G, j = 1, \ldots, N_i\}$. Thus, we obtain $\mathbf{V}_{ij} \subset \mathbf{U}_{ij}$ and $\mathbf{W}_{ij} \subset \mathbf{U}_{ij}$ such that

- $\mathbf{V}_{ij} = (V_{ij,1}, \ldots, V_{ij,q_1})$: q_1-dimensional genes associated with TTP (P-value < 0.001),
- $\mathbf{W}_{ij} = (W_{ij,1}, \ldots, W_{ij,q_2})$: q_2-dimensional genes associated with OS (P-value < 0.001),

where $\mathbf{V}_{ij}$ and $\mathbf{W}_{ij}$ may have common elements since some genes influence both TTP and OS.

If the P-value < 0.001 cutoff is not suitable to data, one can try to find a data-driven cutoff value that optimizes a predictive measure proposed by Matsui (2006). The methodologies and computer programs for obtaining the optimal cutoff in univariate feature selection are available in Emura et al. (2019).

In the initial process of screening genes, we focus on the univariate effect of each gene, ignoring all other effects of genes and covariates. Neither the effect of dependent censoring nor frailty is accounted at this stage.

Then, we construct compound covariates (CCs)

$$
\begin{aligned}
CC_{1,ij} &= \hat{b}_1 V_{ij,1} + \cdots + \hat{b}_{q_1} V_{ij,q_1} \quad \text{(associated with TTP)} \\
CC_{2,ij} &= \hat{c}_1 W_{ij,1} + \cdots + \hat{c}_{q_2} W_{ij,q_2} \quad \text{(associated with OS)}
\end{aligned}
$$

where the weights $\hat{b}_k$ and $\hat{c}_k$ are estimates under the univariate Cox models on the k-th gene, namely, $\hat{b}_k = \arg \max \ell_k(b_k)$, where

$$
\ell_k(b_k) = \sum_{i=1}^{G} \sum_{j=1}^{N_i} \delta_{ij} \left[b_k U_{ij,k} - \log \left(\sum_{\ell \in R_{ij}} \exp(b_k U_{\ell,k}) \right) \right], \quad R_{ij} = \{\ell; T_\ell \geq T_{ij}\},
$$

and $\hat{c}_k = \arg \max \ell_k^*(c_k)$, where

$$
\ell_k^*(c_k) = \sum_{i=1}^{G} \sum_{j=1}^{N_i} \delta_{ij}^* \left[c_k U_{ij,k} - \log \left(\sum_{\ell \in R_{ij}^*} \exp(c_k U_{\ell,k}) \right) \right], \quad R_{ij}^* = \{\ell; T_\ell^* \geq T_{ij}^*\}.
$$

Let $\hat{\mu}_1$ (or $\hat{\mu}_2$) be the sample mean of $CC_{1,ij}$ (or $CC_{2,ij}$). Also, let $\hat{\sigma}_1$ (or $\hat{\sigma}_2$) be the sample SD of $CC_{1,ij}$ (or $CC_{2,ij}$). The standardized values of the compound covariates are fitted to the joint frailty-copula model (Emura et al. 2017; Chap. 3):

$$
\begin{cases}
r_{ij}(t|u_i) = u_i r_0(t) \exp\left(\boldsymbol{\beta}_1' \mathbf{Z}_{1,ij} + \gamma_1 \{ CC_{1,ij} - \hat{\mu}_1 \}/\hat{\sigma}_1 \right) \\
\lambda_{ij}(t|u_i) = u_i^\alpha \lambda_0(t) \exp\left(\boldsymbol{\beta}_2' \mathbf{Z}_{2,ij} + \gamma_2 \{ CC_{2,ij} - \hat{\mu}_2 \}/\hat{\sigma}_2 \right), \\
\Pr(X_{ij} > x, D_{ij} > y | u_i) = C_\theta [S_{Xij}(x|u_i), S_{Dij}(y|u_i)]
\end{cases} \quad (4.1)
$$

where u_i is a frailty term for the i-th study, C_θ is a copula with a parameter θ, $r_0(t) = \mathbf{g}'\mathbf{M}(t)$ and $\lambda_0(t) = \mathbf{h}'\mathbf{M}(t)$ are baseline hazard functions approximated by splines, and $\mathbf{M}(t) = (M_1(t), \ldots, M_5(t))'$ are the M-spline bases (Appendix A). In Eq. (4.1), the survival functions and hazard functions are related through

$$\begin{cases} S_{Xij}(x|u_i) = \exp\left[-u_i R_0(x) \exp(\boldsymbol{\beta}_1' \mathbf{Z}_{1,ij} + \gamma_1\{CC_{1,ij} - \hat{\mu}_1\}/\hat{\sigma}_1)\right], \\ S_{Dij}(y|u_i) = \exp\left[-u_i^{\alpha} \Lambda_0(y) \exp(\boldsymbol{\beta}_2' \mathbf{Z}_{2,ij} + \gamma_2\{CC_{2,ij} - \hat{\mu}_2\}/\hat{\sigma}_2)\right], \end{cases} \quad (4.2)$$

where $R_0(x) = \int_0^x r_0(t)dt$ and $\Lambda_0(y) = \int_0^y \lambda_0(t)dt$. The parameter estimates $(\hat{\eta}, \hat{\theta}, \hat{\boldsymbol{\beta}}_1, \hat{\boldsymbol{\beta}}_2, \hat{\gamma}_1, \hat{\gamma}_2, \hat{\mathbf{g}}, \hat{\mathbf{h}})$ are computed through *jointCox.reg()* in the *joint.Cox* R package (Emura 2019), where $\hat{\eta}$ is an estimate of the heterogeneity parameter $\eta = \mathrm{Var}(u_i)$.

Remarks We apply the standardized version of a compound covariate since the range of $CC_{1,ij}$ (or $CC_{2,ij}$) can be very large if the number q_1 (or q_2) is large. In general, fitting a large covariate value may yield computational difficulties in the joint frailty-copula model.

4.6 The Joint Model with Ridge or Lasso Predictor

In addition to the compound covariate method, a variety of approaches are available to deal with high-dimensional covariates (Bøvelstad et al. 2007). The ridge approach does not involve the preliminary selection of genes, unlike the compound covariate predictor that screens out genes with a P-value threshold. Instead, the ridge approach requires selecting a shrinkage parameter that plays a similar role as the P-value threshold. We should notice that using the whole genes for prediction appears to be uncommon in medical practices, and hence, this approach should be considered with their practical feasibility for clinicians. Nevertheless, as the ridge regression is an accurate and sophisticated statistical prediction tool in gene expression data (Bøvelstad et al. 2007; van Wieringen et al. 2009), it is worth considering this approach.

The ridge approach uses the genes $\mathbf{U}_{ij} = (U_{ij,1}, \ldots, U_{ij,p})$ to construct predictors

$$\begin{aligned} \mathrm{Ridge}_{1,ij} &= \hat{\xi}_1 U_{ij,1} + \cdots + \hat{\xi}_p U_{ij,p} = \hat{\boldsymbol{\xi}}' \mathbf{U}_{ij} \quad \text{(associated with TTP)} \\ \mathrm{Ridge}_{2,ij} &= \hat{\varsigma}_1 U_{ij,1} + \cdots + \hat{\varsigma}_p U_{ij,p} = \hat{\boldsymbol{\varsigma}}' \mathbf{U}_{ij} \quad \text{(associated with OS)} \end{aligned}, $$

where the weights $\hat{\boldsymbol{\xi}}$ and $\hat{\boldsymbol{\varsigma}}$ are the ridge estimates (Bøvelstad et al. 2007). Specifically, with the model $r_{ij}(t) = r_0(t) \exp(\boldsymbol{\xi}' \mathbf{U}_{ij})$ and the data $\{(T_{ij}, \delta_{ij}, \mathbf{U}_{ij}); i = 1, \ldots, G, j = 1, \ldots, N_i\}$, one can calculate $\hat{\boldsymbol{\xi}}$ by applying *optL2(,fold = 5)* in the *penalized* R package (Goeman et al. 2016). Here, the shrinkage parameter is optimized by using the 5-fold cross-validation as indicated in the option "*fold = 5*". Similarly, one can calculate $\hat{\boldsymbol{\varsigma}}$ by the data $\{(T_{ij}^*, \delta_{ij}^*, \mathbf{U}_{ij}); i = 1, \ldots, G, j = 1, \ldots, N_i\}$. Finally, the joint frailty-copula model is fitted as

$$\begin{cases} r_{ij}(t|u_i) = u_i r_0(t) \exp(\boldsymbol{\beta}_1' \mathbf{Z}_{1,ij} + \gamma_1 \mathrm{Ridge}_{1,ij}) \\ \lambda_{ij}(t|u_i) = u_i^{\alpha} \lambda_0(t) \exp(\boldsymbol{\beta}_2' \mathbf{Z}_{2,ij} + \gamma_2 \mathrm{Ridge}_{2,ij}) \\ \Pr(X_{ij} > x, D_{ij} > y|u_i) = C_\theta[S_{Xij}(x|u_i), S_{Dij}(y|u_i)] \end{cases}.$$

The Lasso-based predictors are computed by the command $optL1(,fold = 5)$, which are denoted as

$$\text{Lasso}_{1,ij} = \hat{\xi}_1 U_{ij,1} + \cdots + \hat{\xi}_p U_{ij,p} = \hat{\xi}' \mathbf{U}_{ij} \quad \text{(associated with TTP)}$$
$$\text{Lasso}_{2,ij} = \hat{\varsigma}_1 U_{ij,1} + \cdots + \hat{\varsigma}_p U_{ij,p} = \hat{\varsigma}' \mathbf{U}_{ij} \quad \text{(associated with OS)}$$

Note that some estimated regression coefficients are exactly zero in the Lasso method. Thus, only those genes having nonzero estimates ($\hat{\xi}_k \neq 0$ or $\hat{\varsigma}_k \neq 0$) contribute to the predictors.

Both the ridge and Lasso predictors have strong shrinkage effects on their regression coefficients for a large number p. Consequently, the ranges of the predictors are reduced by the shrinkage effect, which make it possible to fit them without standardization.

4.7 Prediction of Patient-Level Survival Function

The patient-level survival function can be obtained for a new patient not in the samples. We follow the general idea of Matsui et al. (2012) who developed a patient-level survival function using compound covariates.

Let D be OS of the new patient. We wish to predict the survival function of D according to the clinical covariates $\mathbf{Z}_2$ and gene expressions $\mathbf{U}_{ij} = (U_{ij,1}, \ldots, U_{ij,p})$. We define a compound covariate

$$CC_2 = \hat{c}_1 W_1 + \cdots + \hat{c}_{q_2} W_{q_2},$$

using the subset $\mathbf{W} = (W_1, \ldots, W_{q_2}) \subset (U_1, \ldots, U_p)$ obtained from the new patient and the estimate $\hat{c}_k$ under the univariate Cox models on the k-th gene.

We assume that the new patient follows the same probability mechanism as the patients in the samples. That is, the new patient has survival experience following the model (4.2). Since the frailty term is usually unknown for the new patient, we integrate out Eq. (4.2) to estimate the patient-level survival function.

$$\hat{S}(w|\mathbf{Z}_2, CC_2) = \int_0^\infty \exp\left\{-u^\alpha \hat{\Lambda}_0(w) \exp\left(\hat{\boldsymbol{\beta}}'_2 \mathbf{Z}_2 + \hat{\gamma}_2 \frac{CC_2 - \hat{\mu}_2}{\hat{\sigma}_2}\right)\right\} f_{\hat{\eta}}(u) du.$$

The confidence interval (CI) for $\hat{S}(w|\mathbf{Z}_2, CC_2)$ is computed by simulating parameters

$$(\hat{\eta}^{*(m)}, \hat{\theta}^{*(m)}, \hat{\boldsymbol{\beta}}_1^{*(m)}, \hat{\boldsymbol{\beta}}_2^{*(m)}, \hat{\gamma}_1^{*(m)}, \hat{\gamma}_2^{*(m)}, \hat{\mathbf{g}}^{*(m)}, \hat{\mathbf{h}}^{*(m)}), \quad m = 1, 2, \ldots, 500,$$

from a multivariate normal distribution

$(\log(\hat{\eta}^*), \log(\hat{\theta}^*), \hat{\boldsymbol{\beta}}_1^*, \hat{\boldsymbol{\beta}}_2^*, \hat{\gamma}_1^*, \hat{\gamma}_2^*, \log(\hat{\mathbf{g}}^*), \log(\hat{\mathbf{h}}^*))$

$\sim N\Big(\text{Mean} = (\log(\hat{\eta}), \log(\hat{\theta}), \hat{\boldsymbol{\beta}}_1, \hat{\boldsymbol{\beta}}_2, \hat{\gamma}_1, \hat{\gamma}_2, \log(\hat{\mathbf{g}}), \log(\hat{\mathbf{h}})), \text{Covariance} = \Sigma\Big),$

where Σ is the log-scaled covariance matrix of the parameter estimates, which is obtained from the outputs of *jointCox.reg(,convergence.par = TRUE)*. Accordingly, we have simulated patient-level survival functions

$$\hat{S}^{*(m)}(w|\mathbf{Z}_2, \text{CC}_2), \quad m = 1, 2, \ldots, 500.$$

Their 2.5 and 97.5% points give the pointwise 95% CI for the patient-level survival function. Note that the delta method is difficult to use for computing the SE and 95% CI due to a large number of parameters.

4.8 Simulations

We conduct a simulation to compare the compound covariate predictor with three other predictors: (i) the ridge-based predictor, (ii) Lasso-based predictor, and (iii) null predictor. The evaluation criterion is the prediction error (also known as the Brier score), defined as

$$\text{Err}(w) = E[\{\mathbf{I}(D > w) - \hat{S}(w|f(Z, \mathbf{U}))\}^2], \quad w > 0,$$

where Z is a clinical covariate, $\mathbf{U} = (U_1, \ldots, U_p)$ are gene expressions, and $f(\cdot)$ can be $f(Z, \mathbf{U}) = (Z, \text{CC}_2)$, $f(Z, \mathbf{U}) = (Z, \text{Ridge}_2)$, $f(Z, \mathbf{U}) = (Z, \text{Lasso}_2)$, or $f(Z, \mathbf{U}) = (0, 0)$. The expectation $E[\cdot]$ is taken for the distribution of $(D, Z, \mathbf{U})$ given $\hat{S}(w|\cdot)$ (Gerds and Schumacher 2006). We calculate $\text{Err}(w)$ according to the following simulation designs.

4.8.1 Simulation Designs

Let $G = 5$ and $N_i = 200$ for $i = 1, 2, \ldots, 5$. A frailty value u_i follows a gamma distribution with $\eta = 0.5$, and a covariate Z_{ij} follows $N(0, 1)$ truncated between -3 and 3. Gene expressions $\mathbf{U}_{ij} = (U_{ij,1}, \ldots, U_{ij,p})$ with $p = 400$ follow a uniform distribution with mean $= 0$ and SD $= 1$ whose correlation structure is $\text{Corr}(U_{ij,k}, U_{ij,\ell}) = 0.5$ for $1 \le k < l \le 25$ or $26 \le k < l \le 50$; $\text{Corr}(U_{ij,k}, U_{ij,\ell}) = 0$ otherwise. The corresponding coefficients are

$$\boldsymbol{\xi}' = (\underbrace{0.1, \ldots, 0.1}_{\times 25}, \underbrace{-0.1, \ldots, -0.1}_{\times 25}, \underbrace{0, \ldots, 0}_{\times 350}).$$

We generated such gene expressions by the command: $X.pathway(n = 1, p = 400, q1 = 25, q2 = 25)$ using the *compound.Cox* R package (Emura et al. 2019).

Given u_i, Z_{ij}, and $\mathbf{U}_{ij}$, the pair of X_{ij} and D_{ij} were generated from the model

$$
\begin{cases}
r_{ij}(t|u_i) = u_i r_0(t) \exp(1.5 \times Z_{ij} + \boldsymbol{\xi}' \mathbf{U}_{ij}) \ \text{(for } X_{ij}) \\
\lambda_{ij}(t|u_i) = u_i \lambda_0(t) \exp(1.5 \times Z_{ij} + \boldsymbol{\xi}' \mathbf{U}_{ij}) \ \big(\text{for } D_{ij}\big) \\
\Pr(X_{ij} > x, D_{ij} > y|u_i) = [S_{Xij}(x|u_i)^{-\theta} + S_{Dij}(y|u_i)^{-\theta} - 1]^{-1/\theta}
\end{cases},
$$

where $\lambda_0(t) = r_0(t) = 1$ and $\theta = 6$ (Kendall's tau = 0.75). Censoring variables C_{ij} were generated from a uniform distribution on $(0, 5)$ that yielded about 30% censored subjects. The training data consist of $\{(T_{ij}, T_{ij}^*, \delta_{ij}, \delta_{ij}^*, Z_{ij}, \mathbf{U}_{ij}); i = 1, \ldots, 5, j = 1, \ldots, 200\}$.

After fitting the data to the joint frailty-copula model, we calculated the patient-level survival function $\hat{S}(w|\cdot)$. To calculate the prediction error, we independently generated the *test data* $\{(X_{ij}^{\text{Test}}, D_{ij}^{\text{Test}}, Z_{ij}^{\text{Test}}, \mathbf{U}_{ij}^{\text{Test}}); i = 1, \ldots, 5, j = 1, \ldots, 200\}$ using the same algorithms as the training data (with different random seeds). The prediction error was then estimated as

$$
\text{Err}(w) = \frac{1}{1000} \sum_{i=1}^{5} \sum_{j=1}^{200} \left\{ \mathbf{I}(D_{ij}^{\text{Test}} > w) - \hat{S}(w|f(Z_{ij}^{\text{Test}}, \mathbf{U}_{ij}^{\text{Test}}) \right\}^2.
$$

For the null predictor, we used the Kaplan–Meier estimator $\hat{S}(w|\cdot)$ computed by the data $\{(T_{ij}^*, \delta_{ij}^*, U_{ij,k}); i = 1, \ldots, 5, j = 1, \ldots, 200\}$. We report the average of the prediction errors for 50 repetitions.

4.8.2 Simulation Results

Figure 4.1 compares the prediction error curve $\text{Err}(w)$, $0 \leq w \leq 3$, for the four different predictors (null, compound covariate, ridge, and Lasso). The smallest prediction error was achieved by the compound covariate predictor. The Lasso and ridge predictors exhibited very similar prediction errors. The three predictors (compound covariate, ridge, and Lasso) expressed remarkably smaller prediction errors compared to the null predictor.

We explore the reason why the compound covariate is successful. On average, the predictor $CC_2 = \hat{c}_1 W_1 + \cdots + \hat{c}_{q_2} W_{q_2}$ contains $q_2 \approx 50.34$ genes. Hence, the average number of q_2 is close to the number of nonzero coefficients in the population coefficients $\boldsymbol{\xi}$. Figure 4.2 displays P-values for the 400 genes from a single simulation run. We see that 50 P-values are below 0.001, and they exactly correspond to the 50 informative genes. Hence, all the 50 informative genes are selected into $CC_2 = \hat{c}_1 W_1 + \cdots + \hat{c}_{50} W_{50}$.

On average, the Lasso-based predictor had $\{j : \hat{\varsigma}_j \neq 0\} = 62.98$ genes of nonzero coefficients. This implies that the Lasso predictor contains at least 12 non-informative genes (noise genes). In the ridge-based predictor, the coefficients of the

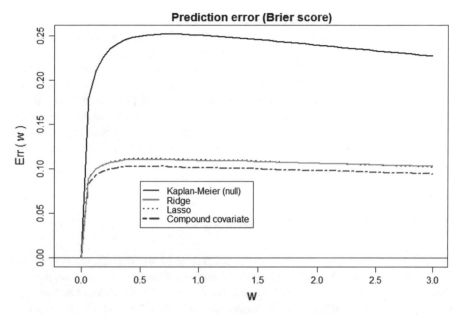

Fig. 4.1   The plots of prediction error with four different prediction methods (averaged for 50 runs)

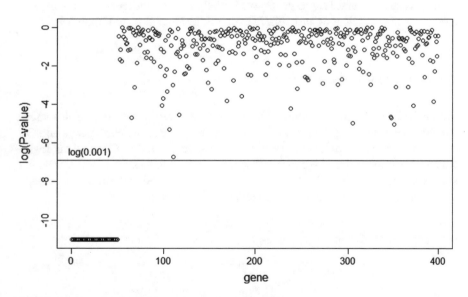

Fig. 4.2   *P*-values for the 400 genes from a single simulation run

50 informative genes are $|\hat{\varsigma}_j| \approx 0.046$ while those of the 350 non-informative genes are $|\hat{\varsigma}_j| \approx 0.001$. Although there are strong shrinkage effects for non-informative genes, they still yield some noises to the ridge-based predictor.

Figure 4.2 also explains the robustness of the compound covariate predictors against the change of the P-value cutoff. The 50 smallest P-values are so small that the selection results are unchanged by decreasing the cutoff P-value of 0.001. If one increases the cutoff P-value from 0.001 to 0.005, two non-informative genes are included in the compound covariate. Since all the 50 informative genes are still kept in the compound covariate, the prediction performance is almost unchanged by the two noise genes.

4.9   Case Study: Ovarian Cancer Data

We performed an IPD meta-analysis on the subset of the ovarian cancer data of Ganzfried et al. (2013) to demonstrate how gene expressions are incorporated into the joint frailty-copula model. Our subset consists of 912 ovarian cancer patients from $G = 4$ different studies (Table 4.1). The detailed process of data extraction is referred to in the bottom of Table 4.1. Across the four studies, 11,756 gene expressions are available. All the expression values are standardized to have mean of 0 and SD of 1 in the patients. Among 11,756 genes, we initially chose a subset consisting of 6056 genes whose coefficient of variation in expression values is greater than 3%.

4.9.1   Compound Covariate

We performed univariate feature selection on the 6056 genes. Figure 4.3 shows the P-values for testing the univariate association between the 6056 genes and OS. Apparently, majority of genes are non-informative to predict OS as their log(P-values) are around zero. We chose 128 genes whose P-values are below 0.001. In a similar fashion, we chose 158 genes univariately associated with time-to-relapse.

Based on the selected genes, we obtained two compound covariates:

$$CC_{1,ij} = (0.249 \times CXCL12_{ij}) + (0.235 \times TIMP2_{ij}) + (0.222 \times PDPN_{ij})$$
$$+ \cdots + (-0.152 \times MMP12_{ij})$$

involving 158 genes (P-value < 0.001 for time-to-relapse), and

$$CC_{2,ij} = (0.237 \times NCOA3_{ij}) + (0.223 \times TEAD1_{ij}) + (0.263 \times YWHAB_{ij})$$
$$+ \cdots + (-0.157 \times KCNH4_{ij}),$$

involving 128 genes (P-value < 0.001 for time-to-death).

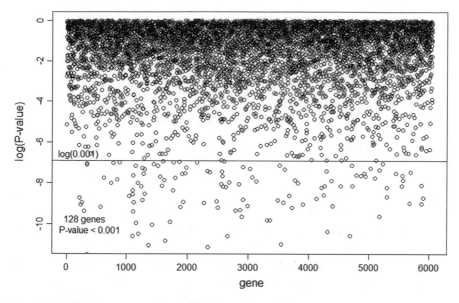

Fig. 4.3 *P*-values for the univariate association between the 6056 genes and OS from the ovarian cancer data. Among them, 128 genes satisfy the *P*-value < 0.001 criterion

In the above CCs, the gene symbols were ordered by their significance. For instance, CXCL12 was the most strongly associated gene for time-to-relapse. The supplementary material of Emura et al. (2018) describes how the genes TIMP2, PDPN, NCOA3, TEAD1, and YWHAB are biologically associated with relapse and death. The means and SDs of the compound covariates are

$$\hat{\mu}_1 = \frac{1}{912} \sum_{i=1}^{4} \sum_{j=1}^{N_i} CC_{1,ij} = 0.338, \quad \hat{\sigma}_1 = \sqrt{\frac{1}{911} \sum_{i=1}^{4} \sum_{j=1}^{N_i} (CC_{1,ij} - \hat{\mu}_1)^2} = 10.468,$$

$$\hat{\mu}_2 = \frac{1}{912} \sum_{i=1}^{4} \sum_{j=1}^{N_i} CC_{2,ij} = 0.222, \quad \hat{\sigma}_2 = \sqrt{\frac{1}{911} \sum_{i=1}^{4} \sum_{j=1}^{N_i} (CC_{2,ij} - \hat{\mu}_2)^2} = 7.894.$$

4.9.2   Fitting the Joint Frailty-Copula Model

In addition to the gene expressions, we have a clinical covariate ($Z_{2,ij} = 0$ vs. $= 1$) on the residual tumour size at surgery (≤ 1 cm vs. >1 cm). The *joint.Cox* R package was applied to fit the data to the joint frailty-copula model as

$$\Pr(X > x, D > y|u) = C_{\hat{\theta}}[\hat{S}_X(x|u), \hat{S}_D(y|u)] = [\hat{S}_X(x|u)^{-\hat{\theta}} + \hat{S}_D(y|u)^{-\hat{\theta}} - 1]^{-1/\hat{\theta}},$$

where $\hat{\theta} = 1.9$ (95%CI: 1.5–2.5), giving Kendall's tau $\hat{\tau} = 0.49$ (95%CI: 0.43–0.55), and

$$\hat{S}_X(x|u) = \exp\left\{-u\hat{R}_0(t)\exp\left(\hat{\gamma}_1\frac{CC_1 - \hat{\mu}_1}{\hat{\sigma}_1}\right)\right\},$$

$$\hat{S}_D(y|u) = \exp\left\{-\hat{\Lambda}_0(t)\exp\left(\hat{\beta}_2 Z_2 + \hat{\gamma}_2\frac{CC_2 - \hat{\mu}_2}{\hat{\sigma}_2}\right)\right\}.$$

Here, the frailty term u appears only for the survival function of time-to-relapse as we set $\alpha = 0$ as the best value. All the regression coefficients in the model were significant (P-value < 0.05). Their relative risks were $\exp(\hat{\gamma}_1) = 1.48\,(95\%\text{CI}: 1.37-1.59)$, $\exp(\hat{\beta}_2) = 1.18\,(95\%\text{CI}: 1.03-1.35)$, and $\exp(\hat{\gamma}_2) = 1.56\,(95\%\text{CI}: 1.43-1.70)$. The heterogeneity parameter was $\hat{\eta} = 0.04\,(95\%\text{CI}: 0.01-0.22)$. The baseline hazard functions are estimated as

$$\hat{r}_0(t) = d\hat{R}_0(t)/dt = 0.85 \times M_1(t) + 2.14 \times M_2(t) + 0 \times M_3(t)$$
$$+ 0.07 \times M_4(t) + 0 \times M_5(t),$$

$$\hat{\lambda}_0(t) = d\hat{\Lambda}_0(t)/dt = 0.17 \times M_1(t) + 1.05 \times M_2(t) + 1.24 \times M_3(t)$$
$$+ 0.27 \times M_4(t) + 0 \times M_5(t),$$

for $t \in [0, 6420]$, where 6420 (days) is the maximum follow-up time.

Appendix B (B.2) provides our R codes to reproduce the fitted values of the above analysis.

4.9.3 Patient-Level Survival Function

To see how the patient-level survival function is predicted, we consider four hypothetical patients (named Patients 1–4) with the following characteristics:

- **Patient 1**: risk genes ($CC_2 = 16$); the residual tumour >1 cm ($Z_2 = 1$),
- **Patient 2**: protective genes ($CC_2 = -16$); the residual tumour ≤ 1 cm ($Z_2 = 0$),
- **Patient 3**: average genes ($CC_2 = 0$); $Z_2 = 1$,
- **Patient 4**: average genes ($CC_2 = 0$); $Z_2 = 0$.

Here, the values of $CC_2 = \pm 16$ are chosen based on a two SD change from the mean such that $\hat{\mu}_2 + 2\hat{\sigma}_2 \approx 16$ and $\hat{\mu}_2 - 2\hat{\sigma}_2 \approx -16$.

Figure 4.4 displays the patient-level survival function for Patients 1–4. Patient 1 has the shortest survival, e.g., the predicted survival probability at 1500 days (about 4 years) is only 15%. In contrast, Patient 2 achieves the longest survival with the

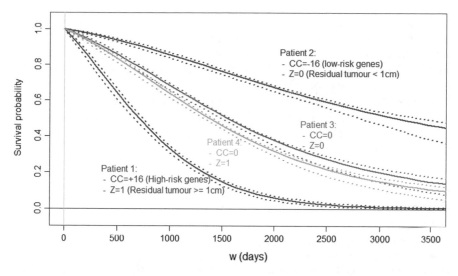

Fig. 4.4 The patient-level survival functions and their 95% CIs (dotted lines)

predicted survival probability 76% at 1500 days. The tight confidence intervals for their predicted survival probabilities confirm that the difference between Patient 1 and Patient 2 is not by chance. However, the difference of survival probabilities between Patient 3 and Patient 4 is less clear.

4.10 Concluding Remarks

To handle high-dimensional covariates, we adopted a simple approach based on Tukey's compound covariate followed by univariate feature selection. We applied the compound covariate predictor to the joint frailty-copula model and developed a patient-level prediction scheme for survival. In our simulations, the compound covariate method showed better predictive ability than the ridge-based or Lasso-based approach. In analysis of ovarian cancer patients, we showed that the developed patient-level survival can classify patients into low, medium, and high-risk groups. However, we recognize the need for validating our prediction formula with an independent validation set of patients before it is widely applied by clinicians.

Our patient-level prediction of OS is based on covariates collected at the study entry time. In the example of the ovarian cancer data, the study entry time refers to the time at surgery where a tumour is surgically removed and its gene expressions and residual tumour size are measured. If necessary, the prediction of OS is updated at each scheduled monitoring date after surgery. Such a dynamic prediction scheme needs a more elaborate formulation than the patient-level survival function considered in this chapter. We shall discuss this topic in details in Chap. 5.

A successful predictor based on gene expressions should not omit informative genes. It is known that omitting informative gene from a predictor has a greater deleterious effect than including non-informative genes (Simon 2005). Thus, it may be difficult to develop a successful predictor based on a small number of genes. For instance, a large number of informative genes are encountered in the lymphoma data reported in Matsui (2006), where the optimized number of genes is 75 or 85. In our illustrative example of ovarian cancer patients, univariate selection yielded 128 genes associated with time-to-death and 158 genes associated with time-to-relapse (P-value < 0.001).

References

Beer DG, Kardia SLR, Huang CC, Giordano TJ, Levin AM et al (2002) Gene-expression profiles predict survival of patients with lung adenocarcinoma. Nat Med 8:816–824

Bickel PJ, Levina E (2004) Some theory for Fisher's linear discriminant function, naive Bayes, and some alternatives when there are many more variables than observations. Bernoulli 10(6):989–1010

Bøvelstad HM, Nygård S, Storvold HL, Aldrin M, Borgan Ø et al (2007) Predicting survival from microarray data—a comparative study. Bioinformatics 23:2080–2087

Chen HY, Yu SL, Chen CH, Chang GC, Chen CY et al (2007) A five-gene signature and clinical outcome in non-small-cell lung cancer. N Engl J Med 356:11–20

Cox DR (1972) Regression models and life-tables (with discussion). J R Stat Soc Series B Stat Methodol 34:187–220

Dudoit S, Fridlyand J, Speed TP (2002) Comparison of discrimination methods for the classification of tumors using gene expression data. J Am Stat Assoc 97(457):77–87

Emura T (2019) joint.Cox: joint frailty-copula models for tumour progression and death in meta-analysis, CRAN

Emura T, Chen YH, Chen HY (2012) Survival prediction based on compound covariate under Cox proportional hazard models. PLoS ONE 7(10):e47627. https://doi.org/10.1371/journal.pone.0047627

Emura T, Nakatochi M, Murotani K, Rondeau V (2017) A joint frailty-copula model between tumour progression and death for meta-analysis. Stat Methods Med Res 26(6):2649–2666

Emura T, Nakatochi M, Matsui S, Michimae H, Rondeau V (2018) Personalized dynamic prediction of death according to tumour progression and high-dimensional genetic factors: meta-analysis with a joint model. Stat Methods Med Res 27(9):2842–2858

Emura T, Matsui S, Chen HY (2019) compound.Cox: univariate feature selection and compound covariate for predicting survival. Comput Methods Programs Biomed 168:21–37

Ganzfried BF, Riester M, Haibe-Kains B, Risch T, Tyekucheva S et al (2013) Curated ovarian data: clinically annotated data for the ovarian cancer transcriptome. Database; Article ID bat013. https://doi.org/10.1093/database/bat013

Gerds TA, Schumacher M (2006) Consistent estimation of the expected Brier score in general survival models with right-censored event times. Biometrical Journal 48(6):1029–1040

Goeman J, Meijer R, Chaturvedi N (2016) penalized: L1 (lasso and fused lasso) and L2 (ridge) penalized estimation in GLMs and in the Cox model, CRAN; version 0.9-47

Lossos IS, Czerwinski DK, Alizadeh AA, Wechser MA, Tibshirani R, Botstein D, Levy R (2004) Prediction of survival in diffuse large-B-cell lymphoma based on the expression of six genes. N Engl J Med 350(18):1828–1837

Matsui S (2006) Predicting survival outcomes using subsets of significant genes in prognostic marker studies with microarrays. BMC Bioinform 7:156

Matsui S, Simon RM, Qu P, Shaughnessy JD, Barlogie B, Crowley J (2012) Developing and validating continuous genomic signatures in randomized clinical trials for predictive medicine. Clin Cancer Res 18(21):6065–6073

Schumacher M, Hollander N, Schwarzer G, Binder H, Sauerbrei W (2012) Prognostic factor studies. In Crowley JJ, Hoering A (ed) Handbook of statistics in clinical oncology, 3rd edn. CRC Press, Boca Raton, pp 415–469

Simon R (2003) Design and analysis of DNA microarray investigations. Springer Science & Business Media, New-York

Simon R (2005) Roadmap for developing and validating therapeutically relevant genomic classifiers. J Clin Oncol 23(29):7332–7341

Tukey JW (1993) Tightening the clinical trial. Control Clin Trials 14:266–285

van Wieringen WN, Kun D, Hampel R, Boulesteix AL (2009) Survival prediction using gene expression data: a review and comparison. Comput Stat Data Anal 53(5):1590–1603

Waldron L, Haibe-Kains B, Culhane AC, Riester M, Ding J et al (2014) Comparative meta-analysis of prognostic gene signatures for late-stage ovarian cancer. J Natl Cancer Inst 106(5):dju049

Wang Y, Klijn JG, Zhang Y, Sieuwerts AM et al (2005) Gene-expression profiles to predict distant metastasis of lymph-node-negative primary breast cancer. The Lancet 365(9460):671–679

Witten DM, Tibshirani R (2010) Survival analysis with high-dimensional covariates. Stat Methods Med Res 19:29–51

Zhao SD, Parmigiani G, Huttenhower C, Waldron L (2014) Más-o-menos: a simple sign averaging method for discrimination in genomic data analysis. Bioinformatics 30(21):3062–3069

Chapter 5
Personalized Dynamic Prediction of Survival

Abstract In the development of patient-tailored therapy, there is a great interest in the dynamic prediction of survival at a certain moment in time (e.g., at a follow-up visit after surgery). This chapter considers dynamic prediction formulas of predicting survival for a cancer patient. The prediction formulas incorporate the genetic and clinical covariates collected on the patient entry as well as the tumour progression history evolving after the entry. We first review the framework of dynamic prediction by introducing prediction formulas, such as the conditional failure function and conditional hazard function. We then demonstrate how the parameters in the prediction formulas are estimated by fitting meta-analytic data to the joint frailty-copula model. For illustration, we apply the dynamic prediction formulas to predict survival for ovarian cancer patients.

Keywords Conditional failure function · Conditional hazard function · Gene expression · Meta-analysis · Ovarian cancer · Personalized medicine · Risk prediction · Semi-competing risks · Tumour progression

5.1 Accurate Prediction of Survival

An important question in survival analysis is whether one can *accurately* predict survival for a cancer patient according to the patient's information. A number of data-driven methods have been developed for predicting survival, e.g., for patients with breast cancer (Gómez et al. 2016; Shukla et al. 2018), ovarian cancer (Yoshihara et al. 2010; Enshaei et al. 2015; Emura et al. 2018), and prostate cancer (Guinney et al. 2017). An accurate survival prediction method allows patients to consider their future and physicians to choose an optimal therapy, constituting a core element of *personalized medicine*. According to its definition, personalized medicine seeks to improve health care by advancing the development of patient-tailored therapy based on genetic information (Schleidgen et al. 2013; Hayes et al. 2014).

Waldron et al. (2014) performed a large-scale meta-analysis on late-stage ovarian cancer patients to examine the prediction performances of 14 published methods based on gene expressions. They concluded that 12 methods demonstrate

© The Author(s), under exclusive license to Springer Nature Singapore Pte Ltd. 2019   77
T. Emura et al., *Survival Analysis with Correlated Endpoints*,
JSS Research Series in Statistics, https://doi.org/10.1007/978-981-13-3516-7_5

their statistical significance for predicting overall survival (i.e., time-to-death) for independent validation data (P-value < 0.05). However, they also noted the modest gain in prediction accuracy (c-index of 0.56–0.60), suggesting the need for further improvement to be of clinical value.

Several ideas for improving the accuracy of prediction are listed below

Combine clinical and genetic information

A number of prognostic models have been developed by applying both clinical and genetic information (Matsui 2006; Binder and Schumacher 2008; Bøvelstad et al. 2009; van Houwelingen and Putter 2011; Matsui et al. 2012; Sun et al. 2018). These studies concluded that the model incorporating both clinical and genetic information leads to better predictive ability than the model including one of them alone. They also concluded that the clinical and genetic covariates are independent predictors for survival. For ovarian cancer patients treated by surgery, the residual tumour size and gene expressions are independent clinical and genetic predictors for overall survival (Yoshihara et al. 2010, 2012; Emura et al. 2018).

Use intermediate events

At study entry, available covariates for a patient would be age, stage, grade, residual tumour size, etc. In addition to these covariates, some intermediate events (e.g., tumour progression) may influence survival during the follow-up. The framework of dynamic prediction (van Houwelingen and Putter 2011) offers prediction formulas that utilize the record of intermediate events occurring after study entry. Throughout this chapter, we shall discuss the theory and application of dynamic prediction.

Use larger training samples to build a prediction formula

This idea is critical when a prediction algorithm involves gene selection (feature selection). The results of the selection are unstable for small training samples and high-dimensional features, which could be alleviated by increasing the sample size (Michiels et al. 2005). Meta-analysis of individual patient data (IPD) is one promising way to stabilize the results. However, there are a few technical issues for performing IPD meta-analyses. The first issue is the heterogeneity between studies, which typically demands random-effects models or frailty models (Burzykowski et al. 2001; Rondeau et al. 2015). The second one is the inconsistent definitions of clinical covariates or inconsistently collected measurements between studies, resulting in the scarcity of reliable covariates in prediction models. This facilitates the need to account for residual dependence (Chap. 3). The joint frailty-copula model is a tailored model to resolve these difficulties in IPD meta-analyses (Emura et al. 2017).

Apply robust statistical methods for selecting genes and calculating a predictor:

Even when the sample size is large, the prediction results still depend on the choices of statistical methods and some tuning parameters. Almost all statistical methods for selecting genes and calculating a predictor are "tuned" versions of Cox's partial likelihood method (Bøvelstad et al. 2007; van Wieringen et al. 2009; Witten and Tibshirani 2010; Emura et al. 2019). Users need to specify a tuning parameter to avoid over-fitting of high-dimensional genetic covariates. The tuning parameter can be the P-value threshold in univariate feature selection or the shrinkage parameter in the penalized partial likelihood method (Bøvelstad et al. 2007). In the analysis of a single endpoint, a tuning parameter is usually optimized for the cross-validated partial likelihood (Matsui 2006; Bøvelstad et al. 2007). However, the partial likelihood is no longer applicable to joint models that demand the full likelihood for estimation. In the sequel, we shall apply the compound covariate method (Chap. 4) to attain a good degree of robustness against the choice of tuning parameters.

5.2 Framework of Dynamic Prediction

Dynamic prediction is a methodology that can utilize the record of intermediate events accumulated before making prediction at time t (van Houwelingen and Putter 2011). For example, tumour progression of a patient may be strongly predictive of the patient's overall survival. However, the intermediate events are not available at the study entry (at time $t = 0$) as they evolve with time. The study entry time ($t = 0$) can be defined in a variety of ways, such as the date of surgery, the date of randomization, and the starting date of chemotherapy. The prediction time $t > 0$ can be one of the scheduled follow-up visits, where a clinician may carry out some examinations for a patient.

Let D be time-to-death and X be time-to-tumour progression (TTP) measured from the study entry. Let $\mathbf{Z}$ be a vector of covariates including both clinical and genetic covariates recorded at the entry. In cancer research, D is more often called overall survival (OS). See Chap. 2 for detailed discussions about OS and TTP. It is assumed that $\mathbf{Z}$ is recorded at time $t = 0$ and does not change over time (time-dependent covariates are not considered). Such covariates are often called *baseline covariates*.

In the traditional survival analysis, prediction of OS is based on the survival function $S(w|\mathbf{Z}) = \Pr(D > w|\mathbf{Z})$ where $w > 0$ is a fixed time period (e.g., 5 years). The survival function aims to predict the vital status (alive or dead) after time w. This prediction scheme shall be called *baseline prediction* since the prediction formula $S(w|\mathbf{Z})$ is constructed with the covariates recorded at time $t = 0$. Since X is not available at time $t = 0$, it is not included in the prediction formula.

The simplest form of dynamic prediction utilizes the conditional survival function, defined as

$$S(t, t + w|\mathbf{Z}) = \Pr(D > t + w|D > t, \mathbf{Z}) = \frac{S(t + w|\mathbf{Z})}{S(t|\mathbf{Z})}.$$

If a patient is surviving at time t, the prediction based on the above conditional survival function is more informative than the baseline prediction.

In dynamic prediction, it is customary to use the *conditional failure function*

$$F(t, t + w|\mathbf{Z}) = \Pr(D \leq t + w|D > t, \mathbf{Z})$$
$$= 1 - \Pr(D > t + w|D > t, \mathbf{Z}),$$
$$= 1 - \frac{S(t + w|\mathbf{Z})}{S(t|\mathbf{Z})}$$

rather than the conditional survival function. The conditioning event $\{D \geq t\}$ means that prediction of survival is meaningful only when a patient is still alive at time $t > 0$. In this sense, the conditional failure function is similar to the hazard function that quantifies the instantaneous risks of death for those who are alive at time $t > 0$. Indeed, the hazard function is related to the conditional failure function through

$$\lambda(t|\mathbf{Z}) = \frac{F(t, t + dw|\mathbf{Z})}{dw} = \left. \frac{dF(t, t + w|\mathbf{Z})}{dw} \right|_{w=0}.$$

In dynamic prediction, a prediction formula is constructed at $t > 0$ so that progression information about X may be available in addition to $\{ D \geq t \}$ and $\mathbf{Z}$. We shall call t as *prediction time*, the time at which a clinician makes a prediction for a patient.

5.2.1 Conditional Failure Function

First, suppose that a patient does not experience tumour progression at time t (i.e., $X > t$). Given that the patient is alive at time t, the conditional probability of death between t and $t + w$ is

$$F(t, t + w|X > t, \mathbf{Z}) = \Pr(D \leq t + w| D > t, X > t, \mathbf{Z}).$$

Second, suppose that a patient experiences tumour progression before time t and that the time of the tumour progression (i.e., $X = x$) is available at time t. Given that the patient is still alive at time t, the conditional probability of death between t and $t + w$ is

$$F(t, t + w|X = x, \mathbf{Z}) = \Pr(D \leq t + w| D > t, X = x, \mathbf{Z}), \quad x \leq t.$$

Tumour progression occurring to a patient may increase his/her probability of death. Thus, one may expect the inequality $F(t, t + w|X = x, \mathbf{Z}) > F(t, t + w|X > t, \mathbf{Z})$ to hold for $w > 0$ (Fig. 5.1). This inequality is usually implied by positive dependence between X and D. Clearly, the equality $F(t, t + w|X = x, \mathbf{Z}) = F(t, t + w|X > t, \mathbf{Z})$ is implied by the conditional independence between X and D given $\mathbf{Z}$.

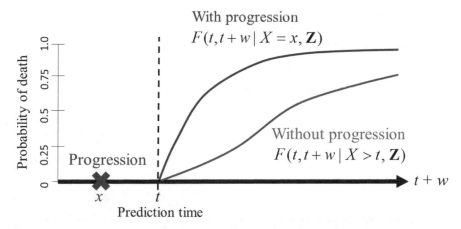

Fig. 5.1 Tumour progression occurring to a patient may increase his/her probability of death. Thus, the inequality $F(t, t + w|X = x, \mathbf{Z}) > F(t, t + w|X > t, \mathbf{Z})$ holds for $w > 0$

The prediction time t should be chosen prospectively. For instance, t can be chosen according to calendar schedule (e.g., every 6 weeks after treatment) prescribed in a clinical trial. This schedule should not be influenced by the health status of a patient or any other reasons that might be informative for survival.

Figure 5.2 demonstrates a dynamic prediction for four hypothetical patients (named Patients 1–4). Patients 1 and 2 have died before time t, so they are excluded from the target for prediction. Patients 3 and 4 are alive at time t, so they are the target for prediction. Patient 3 experiences tumour progression before time t, so the prediction formula incorporates TTP. Patient 4 does not experience tumour progression before time t, so the prediction formula incorporates the information that TTP is greater than time t.

In dynamic prediction, the conditional failure function provides graphical tools to demonstrate the time-varying risks of death. To facilitate the interpretation, one may fix either t or w.

Given w, the conditional failure function is interpreted analogously with the conditional hazard function. It represents how the amount of risk changes over time t. The increasing (decreasing) hazard function typically corresponds to the increasing conditional failure function (decreasing). van Houwelingen and Putter (2011) provide several examples to demonstrate this way of interpreting the conditional failure function.

Given t, the conditional failure function is interpreted analogously with the usual distribution function; it is an increasing function from zero (at $w = 0$) to one (at $w = \infty$). The plot of the conditional failure function against w depicts how the risk of death evolves over time (Mauguen et al. 2013; Emura et al. 2018). See Fig. 5.1.

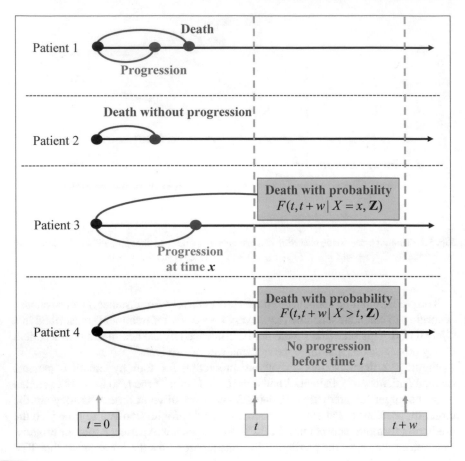

Fig. 5.2 Dynamic prediction of death according to tumour progression. Prediction is not performed for Patients 1 and 2 who have died before time t. Prediction is performed for Patients 3 and 4 according to their tumour progression status observed before time t

5.2.2   *Conditional Hazard Function*

We define the conditional hazard function by letting w to be a small number dw in the conditional failure function. Specifically, we define two conditional hazard functions as

$$\lambda(t|X = x, \mathbf{Z}) = F(t, t + dw|X = x, \mathbf{Z})/dw,$$

$$\lambda(t|X > x, \mathbf{Z}) = F(t, t + dw|X > x, \mathbf{Z})/dw.$$

Dependence between X and D is assessed by the *cross-ratio function* (Oakes 1989)

$$\frac{\lambda(t|X=x, \mathbf{Z})}{\lambda(t|X>x, \mathbf{Z})} = \frac{\Pr(X=x, D=t|\mathbf{Z})\Pr(X>x, D>t|\mathbf{Z})}{\Pr(X=x, D>t|\mathbf{Z})\Pr(X>x, D=t|\mathbf{Z})}, \quad t>0, \quad x>0.$$

The ratio greater than 1 corresponds to positive dependence while the ratio less than 1 corresponds to negative dependence. See Chap. 2 for more details about the cross-ratio function.

The cross-ratio function was originally employed by Clayton (1978) in order to introduce a bivariate survival model that satisfies

$$\lambda(t|X=x, \mathbf{Z}) = (\theta+1)\lambda(t|X>x, \mathbf{Z}), \quad t>0, \quad x>0. \tag{5.1}$$

for some constant $\theta>0$. This is a proportional hazards model for the effect of $\{X=x\}$ relative to the effect of $\{X>x\}$, where the parameter $(\theta+1)$ represents the relative risk. Clayton (1978) introduced a model

$$\Pr(X>x, D>t|\mathbf{Z}) = [S_X(x|\mathbf{Z})^{-\theta} + S_D(t|\mathbf{Z})^{-\theta} - 1]^{-\frac{1}{\theta}}, \quad t>0, \quad x>0,$$

where $S_X(x|\mathbf{Z})$ and $S_D(t|\mathbf{Z})$ are arbitrary continuous survival functions. Equation (5.1) holds true under Clayton's model, irrespective of the forms of $S_X(\cdot|\cdot)$ and $S_D(\cdot|\cdot)$. Clearly, Clayton's model has a copula $C_\theta(v, w) = (v^{-\theta} + w^{-\theta} - 1)^{-1/\theta}$ that is the Clayton copula.

The cross-ratio function was also employed by Day et al. (1997) in the landmark analysis of dynamic prediction. In the context of dynamic prediction, the interest lies in the case of $t \geq x$ since one is concerned with the instantaneous risk of death at time t according to the *previous* tumour progression status at time x. Especially by letting $t=x$, one can consider the effect of the *current* tumour progression status on the instantaneous risk of death at time t. The corresponding relative risk is

$$\frac{\lambda(t|X=t, \mathbf{Z})}{\lambda(t|X>t, \mathbf{Z})}, \quad t>0.$$

This function represents the current effect of tumour progression on survival at time t. By Eq. (5.1), this function is constant under the Clayton model.

The actual formulas for the conditional failure function and conditional hazard function depend on the types of models. van Houwelingen and Putter (2011) adopted the landmark approach based on the conditional Cox model at each prediction time. In recent years there has been a noticeable trend using joint models that account for the dependence between survival and other responses via frailty. Different frailty models have been developed to join different response types (Rizopoulos 2011; Mauguen et al. 2013, 2015; Proust-Lima et al. 2014; Rondeau et al. 2017; Król et al. 2016; Sène et al. 2016). However, these existing frailty models for dynamic prediction have not been adapted to meta-analyses that combine heterogeneous studies. In the sequel, we introduce the joint frailty-copula model (Chap. 3) to construct the prediction formula based on IPD meta-analyses.

5.3   Prediction Formulas Under the Joint Frailty-Copula Model

We need an appropriate statistical model to derive prediction formulas, such as the conditional failure/hazard function. Since we aim to use meta-analytic data collected from heterogeneous studies, we consider a frailty model. Specifically, let $S_X(x|u) = \Pr(X > x|u, \ \mathbf{Z})$ and $S_D(y|u) = \Pr(D > y|u, \ \mathbf{Z})$ be survival functions given an unobserved frailty term u. Here, we use u to represent the unobserved heterogeneity of patients, which is not explained by observed covariates $\mathbf{Z}$. To simplify the presentation, we have suppressed $\mathbf{Z}$ in the notations of $S_X(x|u)$ and $S_D(y|u)$. We impose the assumption that u follows a gamma distribution with a density

$$f_\eta(u) = \frac{1}{\Gamma(1/\eta)\eta^{1/\eta}} u^{\frac{1}{\eta}-1} \exp\left(-\frac{u}{\eta}\right), \qquad u > 0, \quad \eta > 0.$$

The distribution has mean 1 and variance η that represents the degree of heterogeneity. As in Chap. 3, we consider the joint frailty-copula model

$$\Pr(X > x, \ D > y|u, \ \mathbf{Z}) = C_\theta[S_X(x|u), \ S_D(y|u)],$$

where $C_\theta(v, \ w)$ is a copula, and the parameter θ represents the degree of association between TTP and OS.

Following Emura et al. (2018), we divide a prediction formula into two different cases according to the tumour progression status:

Case I *If the patient does not experience tumour progression before time t (i.e., $X > t$), the conditional failure function is*

$$F(t, t + w|X > t, \ \mathbf{Z}) = \Pr(D \le t + w|D > t, \ X > t, \ \mathbf{Z})$$
$$= \frac{\int_0^\infty (C_\theta[S_X(t|u), \ S_D(t|u)] - C_\theta[S_X(t|u), \ S_D(t + w|u)])f_\eta(u)\mathrm{d}u}{\int_0^\infty C_\theta[S_X(t|u), \ S_D(t|u)]f_\eta(u)\mathrm{d}u},$$

and the conditional hazard function is

$$\lambda(t|X > t, \ \mathbf{Z}, \ u) = \lambda_D(t|u)\frac{S_D(t|u)C_\theta^{[0,1]}[S_X(t|u), \ S_D(t|u)]}{C_\theta[S_X(t|u), \ S_D(t|u)]},$$

where $\lambda_D(t|u) = -\partial \log S_D(t|u)/\partial t$, and $C_\theta^{[0,1]}(v, w) = \partial C_\theta(v, w)/\partial w$.

Case II *If the patient experiences tumour progression before time t (i.e., $X = x$, $x \leq t$), the conditional failure function is*

$$F(t, t + w | X = x, \mathbf{Z}) = \Pr(D \leq t + w | D > t, X = x, \mathbf{Z})$$

$$= \frac{\int_0^\infty \left(C_\theta^{[1,0]}[S_X(x|u), \ S_D(t|u)] - C_\theta^{[1,0]}[S_X(x|u), \ S_D(t+w|u)] \right) \lambda_X(x|u) S_X(x|u) f_\eta(u) du}{\int_0^\infty C_\theta^{[1,0]}[S_X(x|u), \ S_D(t|u)] \lambda_X(x|u) S_X(x|u) f_\eta(u) du},$$

where $\lambda_X(x|u) = -\partial \log S_X(x|u)/\partial x$. The conditional hazard function is

$$\lambda(t|X = x, \mathbf{Z}, u) = \lambda_D(t|u) \frac{S_D(t|u) C_\theta^{[1,1]}[S_X(x|u), \ S_D(t|u)]}{C_\theta^{[1,0]}[S_X(x|u), \ S_D(t|u)]},$$

where $C_\theta^{[1,0]}(v, w) = \partial C_\theta(v, w)/\partial v$ and $C_\theta^{[1,1]}(v, w) = \partial^2 C_\theta(v, w)/\partial v \partial w$.

The derivations of these formulas are given in Appendix C. Appendix C also gives the simplified expressions under the independence copula $C(v, w) = vw$ that corresponds to the joint frailty model of Rondeau et al. (2015).

We have defined the conditional hazard functions given the frailty u rather than integrating it out. The reason is to utilize a mathematical relationship

$$\frac{\lambda(t|X = t, \mathbf{Z}, u)}{\lambda(t|X > t, \mathbf{Z}, u)} = R_\theta[S_X(t|u), \ S_D(t|u)],$$

where

$$R_\theta(v, w) = \frac{C_\theta^{[1,1]}(v, w) C_\theta(v, w)}{C_\theta^{[1,0]}(v, w) C_\theta^{[0,1]}(v, w)}$$

is the cross-ratio function for the copula (Chap. 2). Under the Clayton copula $C_\theta(v, w) = (v^{-\theta} + w^{-\theta} - 1)^{-1/\theta}$, the cross-ratio function becomes $R_\theta(v, w) = 1 + \theta$ that is interpreted as the relative risk of $\{X = t\}$ versus $\{X > t\}$. Some other copulas also induce simple mathematical forms of $R_\theta(v, w)$ (Chap. 2).

To perform dynamic prediction on the basis of the conditional hazard functions, clinicians need to specify the unobserved frailty u. They may choose $u = 1$ which corresponds to the prediction for the average patient. Some sensitivity analysis on the range of $1 - 2\sqrt{\eta} \leq u \leq 1 + 2\sqrt{\eta}$ might also be helpful.

5.4   Estimating Prediction Formulas

Before performing dynamic prediction for a *new* patient, all the unknown parameters in the prediction formulas must be estimated by a training dataset. The new patient refers to a hypothetical patient who is not included in the training dataset. We assume that the survival outcome has not been observed for the new patient, but the baseline covariates $\mathbf{Z} = (\mathbf{Z}_1, \mathbf{Z}_2, \mathrm{CC}_1, \mathrm{CC}_2)$ have been recorded

- $\mathbf{Z}_1$: p_1 clinical covariates associated with TTP,
- $\mathbf{Z}_2$: p_2 clinical covariates associated with OS,
- $\mathrm{CC}_1 = w_1 V_1 + \cdots + w_{q1} V_{q1}$: compound covariate predictor for TTP,
- $\mathrm{CC}_2 = \varpi_1 W_1 + \cdots + \varpi_{q2} W_{q2},$: compound covariate predictor for OS,

where $(V_1, \ldots, V_{q1})$ are q_1 gene expressions associated with TTP, $(W_1, \ldots, W_{q2})$ are q_2 gene expressions associated with OS, where the weights w_k and ϖ_k are determined by the training dataset. Assume that the gene expressions are standardized to have mean $= 0$ and SD $= 1$. A method of selecting q_1 (or q_2) genes and computing w_k (ϖ_k) is detailed in Chap. 4.

By fitting a training dataset to the joint frailty-copula model, one can estimate survival functions for TTP and OS, respectively, as

$$\hat{S}_X(t|u) = \exp\left\{ -u\hat{R}_0(t) \exp\left(\hat{\boldsymbol{\beta}}_1' \mathbf{Z}_1 + \hat{\gamma}_1 \frac{\mathrm{CC}_1 - \hat{\mu}_1}{\hat{\sigma}_1} \right) \right\},$$

$$\hat{S}_D(t|u) = \exp\left\{ -u^\alpha \hat{\Lambda}_0(t) \exp\left(\hat{\boldsymbol{\beta}}_2' \mathbf{Z}_2 + \hat{\gamma}_2 \frac{\mathrm{CC}_2 - \hat{\mu}_2}{\hat{\sigma}_2} \right) \right\},$$

where $\hat{R}_0(t) = \int_0^t \hat{r}_0(x)\mathrm{d}x$ and $\hat{\Lambda}_0(t) = \int_0^t \hat{\lambda}_0(x)\mathrm{d}x$ are estimated baseline hazard functions, and $(\hat{\theta}, \hat{\eta}, \hat{\boldsymbol{\beta}}_1, \hat{\boldsymbol{\beta}}_2, \hat{\gamma}_1, \hat{\gamma}_2, \hat{r}_0, \hat{\lambda}_0)$ are parameter estimates, and $\hat{\mu}_1$ (or $\hat{\mu}_2$) is the mean of CC_1 (or CC_2), and $\hat{\sigma}_1$ (or $\hat{\sigma}_2$) is the SD of CC_1 (or CC_2); the details are referred to Chap. 4. The baseline hazard functions are estimated by $\hat{r}_0(t) = \hat{\mathbf{g}}'\mathbf{M}(t)$ and $\hat{\lambda}_0(t) = \hat{\mathbf{h}}'\mathbf{M}(t)$, where $\mathbf{M}(t) = (M_1(t), \ldots, M_5(t))'$ are the cubic M-spline basis functions (Chap. 3; Appendix A).

These estimates can be applied to compute the conditional failure/hazard functions. For instance, we compute the conditional failure functions

$$\hat{F}(t, t+w|X > t, \mathbf{Z})$$
$$= \frac{\int_0^\infty \left(C_{\hat{\theta}}[\hat{S}_X(t|u), \hat{S}_D(t|u)] - C_{\hat{\theta}}[\hat{S}_X(t|u), \hat{S}_D(t+w|u)] \right) f_{\hat{\eta}}(u)\mathrm{d}u}{\int_0^\infty C_{\hat{\theta}}[\hat{S}_X(t|u), \hat{S}_D(t|u)] f_{\hat{\eta}}(u)\mathrm{d}u},$$

$$\hat{F}(t, t+w|X = x, \mathbf{Z})$$
$$= \frac{\int_0^\infty \left(C_{\hat{\theta}}^{[1,0]}[\hat{S}_X(x|u), \hat{S}_D(t|u)] - C_{\hat{\theta}}^{[1,0]}[\hat{S}_X(x|u), S_D(t+w|u)] \right) \hat{\lambda}_X(x|u)\hat{S}_X(x|u)f_{\hat{\eta}}(u)\mathrm{d}u}{\int_0^\infty C_{\hat{\theta}}^{[1,0]}[\hat{S}_X(x|u), \hat{S}_D(t|u)] \hat{\lambda}_X(x|u)\hat{S}_X(x|u)f_{\hat{\eta}}(u)\mathrm{d}u}.$$

The confidence interval (CI) is computed by a simulation method of Sect. 4.7 in Chap. 4.

Estimates for the conditional hazard $\lambda(t|\cdot)$ are obtained in a similar way.

Remarks The spline basis functions $\mathbf{M}(t)$ are defined on $t \in [\xi_1, \xi_3]$, where ξ_1 is the smallest value of TTP and ξ_3 is the largest value of OS in the training dataset. This implies that the values of $\hat{S}_X(t|u)$ and $\hat{S}_D(t|u)$ are defined if $t \in [\xi_1, \xi_3]$. Accordingly, the values of $\hat{F}(t, t + w|\cdot)$ is defined if both $t \in [\xi_1, \xi_3]$ and $t + w \in [\xi_1, \xi_3]$ hold. If $t < \xi_1$ or $t + w > \xi_3$, the values of $\hat{F}(t, t + w|\cdot)$ are undefined.

5.5 Case Study: Ovarian Cancer Data

We use the data of Ganzfried et al. (2013) to demonstrate the dynamic prediction formulas under the joint frailty-copula model. The data consist of 912 ovarian cancer patients (American, Australian, and Japanese patients) from $G = 4$ studies. The endpoints of interest are time-to-relapse and time-to-death, referred to as TTP and OS, respectively. A large number of gene expressions are available as prognostic factors for TTP and OS. The data is summarized in Table 4.1 of Chap. 4.

As in Chap. 4, we construct compound covariates

$$\mathrm{CC}_1 = (0.249 \times CXCL12) + (0.235 \times TIMP2) + (0.222 \times PDPN)$$
$$+ \cdots + (-0.152 \times MMP12),$$

involving 158 genes (*P*-value < 0.001 for TTP), and

$$\mathrm{CC}_2 = (0.237 \times NCOA3) + (0.223 \times TEAD1) + (0.263 \times YWHAB)$$
$$+ \cdots + (-0.157 \times KCNH4),$$

involving 128 genes (*P*-value < 0.001 for OS).

Here, gene expressions (e.g., *CXCL12*) are standardized to have mean $= 0$ and SD $= 1$ in the 912 patients. The fitted joint frailty-copula model is

$$\Pr(X > x, \ D > y|u) = C_{\hat{\theta}}[\hat{S}_X(x|u), \ \hat{S}_D(y|u)] = [\hat{S}_X(x|u)^{-\hat{\theta}} + \hat{S}_D(y|u)^{-\hat{\theta}} - 1]^{-1/\hat{\theta}},$$

where $\hat{\theta} = 1.9$ (Kendall's tau $\hat{\tau} = 0.49$),

$$\hat{S}_X(x|u) = \exp\left\{-u\hat{R}_0(t)\exp\left(\hat{\gamma}_1\frac{\mathrm{CC}_1 - \hat{\mu}_1}{\hat{\sigma}_1}\right)\right\},$$
$$\hat{S}_D(y|u) = \exp\left\{-\hat{\Lambda}_0(t)\exp\left(\hat{\beta}_2 Z_2 + \hat{\gamma}_2\frac{\mathrm{CC}_2 - \hat{\mu}_2}{\hat{\sigma}_2}\right)\right\},$$

where Z_2 is a clinical covariate (0 or 1) on the residual tumour size at surgery ($\leq$ 1 cm or > 1 cm). The estimates are $\hat{\gamma}_1 = 0.39$, $\hat{\beta}_2 = 0.16$, $\hat{\gamma}_2 = 0.44$, $\hat{\mu}_1 = 0.338$, $\hat{\sigma}_1 = 10.468$, $\hat{\mu}_2 = 0.222$, $\hat{\sigma}_2 = 7.894$,

$$\hat{r}_0(t) = d\hat{R}_0(t)/dt$$
$$= 0.85 \times M_1(t) + 2.14 \times M_2(t) + 0 \times M_3(t) + 0.07 \times M_4(t) + 0 \times M_5(t),$$

$$\hat{\lambda}_0(t) = d\hat{\Lambda}_0(t)/dt$$
$$= 0.17 \times M_1(t) + 1.05 \times M_2(t) + 1.24 \times M_3(t) + 0.27 \times M_4(t) + 0 \times M_5(t),$$

for $t \in [0, \ 6420]$, where 6420 (days) is the maximum follow-up time. The heterogeneity parameter is $\text{Var}(u_i) = \hat{\eta} = 0.04$. Although models including more covariates could be considered, they do not improve the above model in terms of its predictive ability. The R codes given in B2 of Appendix B produce the fitted values.

We use the *joint.Cox* R package (Emura 2019) to perform dynamic prediction on two hypothetical patients with the following baseline covariates

- **Patient 1**: risk genes ($CC_1 = 10$, $CC_2 = 10$)[1]; residual tumour > 1 cm ($Z_2 = 1$).
- **Patient 2**: protective genes ($CC_1 = -10$, $CC_2 = -10$); residual tumour $\leq$ 1 cm ($Z_2 = 0$).

For instance, one can compute the conditional failure function $\hat{F}(t, \ t+w|X = x, \ \mathbf{Z})$ for Patient 2 with $t = 1000$, $t + w < 6420$, and $x = 600$ using the following codes:

---

[1]To compute CC_1 for a real patient, one needs to know his/her 158 gene expressions. We have omitted this process to simplify the presentation. $CC_1 = 10$ is about a one SD change from the mean of CC_1. The same remarks apply to CC_2.

```
library(joint.Cox)
gamma1=0.39 # coefficient for CC1
beta2=0.16 # coefficient for residual tumour
gamma2=0.44 # coefficient for CC2
theta=1.9 # copula parameter
eta=0.04 # frailty parameter
g=c(0.85, 2.14, 0, 0.07, 0) # hazard for TTP
h=c(0.17, 1.05, 1.24, 0.27, 0) # hazard for OS
lower=0 ### lower limit of t ###
upper=6420 #### upper limit of t+w ###
mu1=0.338 # mean of CC1
SD1=10.468 # SD of CC1
mu2=0.222 # mean of CC2
SD2=7.894 # SD of CC2
```

Parameters in the model

```
time=1000
w_num=20
widths=seq(0,upper-time,length=w_num)
```

Prediction time

```
#### Patient 2 ####
CC1=-10;CC2=-10;Z2=0
X=600 ### relapse at 600 days ###
```

Patient information

```
F.prediction(time=time,width=widths,
            Z1=(CC1-mu1)/SD1, Z2=c((CC2-mu2)/SD2,Z2), X=X,
            beta1=gamma1, beta2=c(beta2,gamma2), eta=eta, theta=theta, alpha=0,
            g=g, h=h, lower, upper, Fplot=TRUE)
```

Below are the outputs

```
> F.prediction(time=time, width=widths,
+        Z1=(CC1-mu1)/SD1, Z2=c((CC2-mu2)/SD2,Z2), X=X,
+        beta1=gamma1, beta2=c(beta2, gamma2), eta=eta, theta=theta, alpha=0,
+        g=g, h=h, lower, upper, Fplot=TRUE)
           t        w     X          F
 [1,] 1000     0.0000   600  0.0000000
 [2,] 1000   285.2632   600  0.1949799
 [3,] 1000   570.5263   600  0.3774276
 [4,] 1000   855.7895   600  0.5359442
 [5,] 1000  1141.0526   600  0.6646969
 [6,] 1000  1426.3158   600  0.7633172
 [7,] 1000  1711.5789   600  0.8353011
 [8,] 1000  1996.8421   600  0.8859373
 [9,] 1000  2282.1053   600  0.9206477
[10,] 1000  2567.3684   600  0.9440686
[11,] 1000  2852.6316   600  0.9597602
[12,] 1000  3137.8947   600  0.9702692
[13,] 1000  3423.1579   600  0.9773336
[14,] 1000  3708.4211   600  0.9821059
[15,] 1000  3993.6842   600  0.9853377
[16,] 1000  4278.9474   600  0.9875151
[17,] 1000  4564.2105   600  0.9889508
[18,] 1000  4849.4737   600  0.9898454
[19,] 1000  5134.7368   600  0.9903263
[20,] 1000  5420.0000   600  0.9904741
```

Figure 5.3 displays the conditional failure functions for Patient 1 and Patient 2. At the prediction time $t = 500$ (days), Patient 1 has higher predicted probabilities of death due to the unfavourable baseline covariates, compared to Patient 2. Here, we have assumed that, at the prediction time $t = 500$ (days), both Patient 1 and Patient 2 are relapse-free. To see how these predictions change as time passes, we assume that Patient 2 experiences relapse at $x = 600$ (days), but Patient 1 is still relapse-free at the time $t = 1000$ (days). Then, the predicted probability of death for Patient 2 gets higher than that for Patient 1. This risk inversion explains that the occurrence of relapse is a stronger risk factor than the unfavourable influence of baseline covariates.

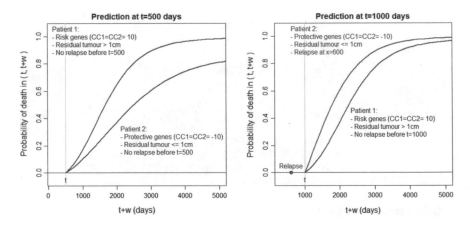

Fig. 5.3 The conditional failure functions computed for two patients

Figure 5.4 displays the conditional hazard function with relapse ($\hat{\lambda}(t|X = t, \mathbf{Z}, u)$) and that without relapse ($\hat{\lambda}(t|X > t, \mathbf{Z}, u)$) at $u = 1$. Since we apply the Clayton copula, the fitted model meets the following proportional hazards relationship

$$\hat{\lambda}(t|X = t, \mathbf{Z}, u) = (1 + \hat{\theta})\hat{\lambda}(t|X > t, \mathbf{Z}, u) = 2.9\hat{\lambda}(t|X > t, \mathbf{Z}, u).$$

Hence, the occurrence of relapse increases the risk of death by almost three times. Figure 5.4 graphically exhibits this relationship. Patient 1 has higher hazard rates of death than Patient 2 due to the unfavourable baseline covariates. The hazard rate for Patient 2 is quite stable and slowly decreasing, irrespective of the relapse status. Patient 2 has fairly good prognosis if relapse does not occur or tumour progression is suppressed during the follow-up (blue line in Fig. 5.4).

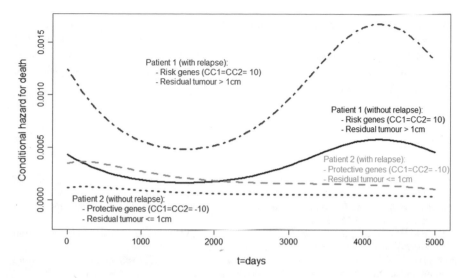

Fig. 5.4 The conditional hazard functions computed for two patients

5.6 Discussions

This chapter has introduced the ideas of dynamic prediction and their implementation under the joint frailty-copula model. We have used the publicly available data on 912 ovarian cancer patients to establish the prediction formulas for overall survival. In addition to the clinical and genetic covariates, the prediction formulas can utilize the record of tumour progression events occurring before the time of prediction, where a copula is used to link the association between OS and TTP. The use of tumour progression information has not been considered in most of the available prediction formulas for ovarian cancer patients, which applied the traditional Cox regression models with clinical covariates and genetic covariates (Tothill et al. 2008; Yoshihara et al. 2010, 2012; Waldron et al. 2014).

Clinicians may use the R codes in Sect. 5.5 to perform prognostic analysis of a surgically treated ovarian cancer patient. Clinicians first enter the following items:

- Prediction time (e.g., **time = 1000** days after surgery),
- Time of tumour progression (e.g., **X = 600** days),
- Residual tumour size (e.g., **Z2 = 0** for residual tumour ≤ 1 cm),
- CCs (e.g., **CC1 = −10** and **CC2 = −10**). They are set as **CC1 = 0** and **CC2 = 0** if no information is available for gene expressions.

Then, the codes automatically produce the predicted probability of death in the next w years.

Emura et al. (2018) performed a leave-one-out cross-validation on the 912 patients to estimate the prediction error of the dynamic prediction formulas. This validation step follows the guideline given by Simon (2005), where both the selection of genes and the estimation of dynamic prediction formulas should be performed without the single left-out sample. Their cross-validation has demonstrated the benefit of using the dynamic prediction formula. However, before the dynamic prediction formulas are applied in clinical practice, an independent validation set may be employed to further assess the prediction ability.

References

Binder H, Schumacher M (2008) Allowing for mandatory covariates in boosting estimation of sparse high-dimensional survival models. BMC Bioinform 9(1):14

Bøvelstad HM, Nygård S, Borgan Ø (2009) Survival prediction from clinico-genomic models—a comparative study. BMC Bioinform 10(1):1

Bøvelstad HM, Nygård S, Storvold HL, Aldrin M, Borgan Ø et al (2007) Predicting survival from microarray data—a comparative study. Bioinformatics 23:2080–2087

Burzykowski T, Molenberghs G, Buyse M, Geys H, Renard D (2001) Validation of surrogate end points in multiple randomized clinical trials with failure time end points. Appl Stat 50(4):405–422

Clayton DG (1978) A model for association in bivariate life tables and its application in epidemiological studies of familial tendency in chronic disease incidence. Biometrika 65(1):141–151

Day R, Bryant J, Lefkopoulou M (1997) Adaptation of bivariate frailty models for prediction, with application to biological markers as prognostic indicators. Biometrika 84(1):45–56

Emura T (2019). joint.Cox: joint frailty-copula models for tumour progression and death in meta-analysis, CRAN

Emura T, Matsui S, Chen HY (2019) compound.Cox: univariate feature selection and compound covariate for predicting survival. Comput Methods Programs Biomed 168:21–37

Emura T, Nakatochi M, Murotani K, Rondeau V (2017) A joint frailty-copula model between tumour progression and death for meta-analysis. Stat Methods Med Res 26(6):2649–2666

Emura T, Nakatochi M, Matsui S, Michimae H, Rondeau V (2018) Personalized dynamic prediction of death according to tumour progression and high-dimensional genetic factors: meta-analysis with a joint model. Stat Methods Med Res 27(9):2842–2858

Enshaei A, Robson CN, Edmondson RJ (2015) Artificial intelligence systems as prognostic and predictive tools in ovarian cancer. Ann Surg Oncol 22(12):3970–3975

Ganzfried BF, Riester M, Haibe-Kains B, Risch T, Tyekucheva S et al (2013). Curated ovarian data: clinically annotated data for the ovarian cancer transcriptome, Database; Article ID bat013: https://doi.org/10.1093/database/bat013

Guinney J, Wang T, Laajala TD, Winner KK et al (2017) Prediction of overall survival for patients with metastatic castration-resistant prostate cancer: development of a prognostic model through a crowdsourced challenge with open clinical trial data. Lancet Oncol 18(1):132–142

Gómez I, Ribelles N, Franco L, Alba E, Jerez JM (2016) Supervised discretization can discover risk groups in cancer survival analysis. Comput Methods Programs Biomed 136:11–19

Hayes DF, Markus HS, Leslie RD, Topol EJ (2014) Personalized medicine: risk prediction, targeted therapies and mobile health technology. BMC Med 12(1):37

Król A, Ferrer L, Pignon JP, Proust-Lima C, Ducreux M et al (2016) Joint model for left-censored longitudinal data, recurrent events and terminal event: Predictive abilities of tumor burden for cancer evolution with application to the FFCD 2000–05 trial. Biometrics 72(3):907–916

Matsui S (2006) Predicting survival outcomes using subsets of significant genes in prognostic marker studies with microarrays. BMC Bioinform 7:156

Matsui S, Simon RM, Qu P, Shaughnessy JD, Barlogie B, Crowley J (2012) Developing and validating continuous genomic signatures in randomized clinical trials for predictive medicine. Clin Cancer Res 18(21):6065–6073

Mauguen A, Rachet B, Mathoulin-Pélissier S, Lawrence GM, Siesling S et al (2015) Validation of death prediction after breast cancer relapses using joint models. BMC Med Res Methodol 15(1):27

Mauguen A, Rachet B, Mathoulin-Pélissier S, MacGrogan G, Laurent A, Rondeau V (2013) Dynamic prediction of risk of death using history of cancer recurrences in joint frailty models. Stat Med 32(30):5366–5380

Michiels S, Koscielny S, Hill C (2005) Prediction of cancer outcome with microarrays: a multiple random validation strategy. The Lancet 365(9458):488–492

Oakes D (1989) Bivariate survival models induced by frailties. J Am Stat Assoc 84:487–493

Proust-Lima C, Séne M, Taylor JM, Jacqmin-Gadda H (2014) Joint latent class models for longitudinal and time-to-event data: a review. Stat Methods Med Res 23(1):74–90

Rizopoulos D (2011) Dynamic predictions and prospective accuracy in joint models for longitudinal and time-to-event data. Biometrics 67(3):819–829

Rondeau V, Mauguen A, Laurent A, Berr C, Helmer C (2017) Dynamic prediction models for clustered and interval-censored outcomes: investigating the intra-couple correlation in the risk of dementia. Stat Methods Med Res 26(5):2168–2183

Rondeau V, Pignon JP, Michiels S (2015) A joint model for dependence between clustered times to tumour progression and deaths: a meta-analysis of chemotherapy in head and neck cancer. Stat Methods Med Res 24(6):711–729

Schleidgen S, Klingler C, Bertram T, Rogowski WH, Marckmann G (2013) What is personalized medicine: sharpening a vague term based on a systematic literature review. BMC Medical Ethics 14(1):55

Sène M, Taylor JM, Dignam JJ, Jacqmin-Gadda H, Proust-Lima C (2016) Individualized dynamic prediction of prostate cancer recurrence with and without the initiation of a second treatment: development and validation. Stat Methods Med Res 25(6):2972–2991

Shukla N, Hagenbuchner M, Win KT, Yang J (2018) Breast cancer data analysis for survivability studies and prediction. Comput Method Program Biomed 155:199–208

Simon R (2005) Roadmap for developing and validating therapeutically relevant genomic classifiers. J Clin Oncol 23(29):7332–7341

Sun D, Li A, Tang B, Wang M (2018) Integrating genomic data and pathological images to effectively predict breast cancer clinical outcome. Comput Method Program Biomed 161:45–53

Tothill RW, Tinker AV, George J, Brown R et al (2008) Novel molecular subtypes of serous and endometrioid ovarian cancer linked to clinical outcome. Clin Cancer Res 14(16):5198–5208

Yoshihara K, Tajima A, Yahata T, Kodama S, Fujiwara H et al (2010) Gene expression profile for predicting survival in advanced-stage serous ovarian cancer across two independent datasets. PLoS ONE 5(3):e9615

Yoshihara K, Tsunoda T, Shigemizu D, Fujiwara H, Hatae M et al (2012) High-risk ovarian cancer based on 126-gene expression signature is uniquely characterized by downregulation of antigen presentation pathway. Clin Cancer Res 18(5):1374–1385

van Houwelingen HC, Putter H (2011) Dynamic prediction in clinical survival analysis. CRC Press, New York

van Wieringen WN, Kun D, Hampel R, Boulesteix AL (2009) Survival prediction using gene expression data: a review and comparison. Comput Stat Data Anal 53(5):1590–1603

Waldron L, Haibe-Kains B, Culhane AC, Riester M, Ding J et al. (2014). Comparative meta-analysis of prognostic gene signatures for late-stage ovarian cancer. J Natl Cancer Inst 106(5):dju049

Witten DM, Tibshirani R (2010) Survival analysis with high-dimensional covariates. Stat Methods Med Res 19:29–51

Chapter 6
Future Developments

Abstract This chapter collects additional remarks on the previous chapters and several open problems for future research. This might help find research topics for students and researchers.

Keywords Compound covariate · Dependent truncation · Interaction · Kendall's τ · Left truncation · Meta-analysis · Recurrent event · Surrogate endpoint

6.1 Recurrent Events Data

The joint frailty-copula model of Chap. 3 can be applicable to analyze recurrent events data if event times are measured in the gap timescale (Emura et al. 2017; Li et al. 2019). Under the recurrent event setting, the interpretation of the joint frailty-copula model is substantially different from the meta-analytic setting of Chap. 3. First, the frailty term represents the effect of unmeasured covariates at patient-level. Thus, this frailty introduces patient-level dependence among recurrences, as well as patient-level dependence between recurrences and death. Second, copulas describe the residual dependence due to unmeasured recurrence-specific covariates. That is, even after covariates and a frailty term are given, a pair of gap time and death time is still dependent. This dependence would be weakened if one could obtain a sufficient amount of recurrence-specific covariates in each recurrence step j (Li et al. 2019).

For instance, Emura et al. (2017) analyzed $G = 403$ patients with colorectal cancer who had operations in a hospital in Spain. The data was originally studied by González et al. (2005) and was made available in R *frailty pack* package (Rondeau and Gonzalez 2005). The patients are followed-up from the date of surgery to either the study end or the time of death whichever comes first. During the follow-up, patients may have several readmissions (recurrences) related to colorectal cancer. The number of recurrences varies from 0 to 22. The results of fitting the joint frailty-copula model under the Clayton copula show that there exists weak residual dependence between readmission and death (Kendall's $\tau = 0.22$, 95%CI: $0.14-0.31$). The reason for residual dependence may be the use of the same set of covariates for all the recurrence steps. This residual dependence could be removed, for instance, by incorporating time-dependent covariates, which are updated at the last discharge date. In the absence of such covariates, the joint frailty-copula model can capture the residual dependence.

As pointed out by Li et al. (2019), the method of Emura et al. (2017) imposes some memoryless or Markov assumption in order to transform the likelihood function from the meta-analytic data to the recurrent event data. This makes it difficult to justify the validity of the likelihood function used in Emura et al. (2017) for recurrent event data. The likelihood derived Li et al. (2019) may resolve these issues. Besides the proposal of Li et al. (2019), there seem to be a few alternative ways to model dependence among recurrent gap times and times to death. For instance, one can consider a copula-based Markov chain for serial dependence between recurrent gap times and another copula for dependence between the first recurrent gap time and time to death.

6.2   Kendall's τ in Meta-Analysis

Kendall's τ is a widely used measure of dependence between two endpoints. For instance, medical researchers have used Kendall's τ between time-to-tumour progression (TTP) and overall survival (OS) to assess the quality TTP as a surrogate endpoint for OS at individual-level (Burzykowski et al. 2001; Rotolo et al. 2018). See also real data examples in Chaps. 3–5 that use Kendall's τ between TTP and OS.

Let us reconsider the definition of Kendall's τ in a meta-analysis that combines several different studies. In Chaps. 3–5 and in Burzykowski et al. (2001), Kendall's τ is actually be regarded as an "individual-level Kendall's τ" as it is defined given a frailty value.

In the following, two versions of Kendall's τ shall be defined with and without a given frailty value. Let X be TTP, D be OS, and U be frailty. Suppose that (X, D, U) has the joint density $f(x, y, u) = f(x, y|u)f(u)$.

The *individual-level Kendall τ* is defined as

$$\tau^{\text{Ind}}(u) = \Pr\{(X_2 - X_1)(D_2 - D_1) > 0|u\} - \Pr\{(X_2 - X_1)(D_2 - D_1) < 0|u\},$$

where $(X_i, D_i) \sim f(x, y|u)$, $i = 1$ and 2, are independent pairs.

The *population-level Kendall τ* is defined as

$$\tau^{\text{Pop}} = \Pr\{(X_2 - X_1)(D_2 - D_1) > 0\} - \Pr\{(X_2 - X_1)(D_2 - D_1) < 0\},$$

where $(X_i, D_i, U_i) \sim f(x, y, u)$, $i = 1$ and 2, are independent pairs.

The population-level Kendall τ involves a double integration on two frailty variables such that

$$
\begin{aligned}
\tau^{\text{Pop}} &= E_{U_1 U_2}[\Pr\{(X_2 - X_1)(D_2 - D_1) > 0 | U_1, U_2\} - \Pr\{(X_2 - X_1)(D_2 - D_1) < 0 | U_1, U_2\}] \\
&= 2 E_{U_1 U_2}[\Pr\{(X_2 - X_1)(D_2 - D_1) > 0 | U_1, U_2\} - 1] \\
&= 2 E_{U_1 U_2}[\Pr\{X_2 < X_1, D_2 < D_1 | U_1, U_2\} + \Pr\{X_2 > X_1, D_2 > D_1 | U_1, U_2\} - 1] \\
&= 2 E_{U_1 U_2}\left[\iint S(x, y|U_1) f(x, y|U_2)\mathrm{d}x\mathrm{d}y + \iint S(x, y|U_2) f(x, y|U_1)\mathrm{d}x\mathrm{d}y \right] - 1.
\end{aligned}
$$

Rondeau et al. (2015) showed that the above expression depends only on the frailty distribution under their joint frailty model. Under the joint frailty-copula models, the expression may also depend on the copula. It is important to note that

$$
\tau^{\text{Pop}} \neq E\left[\tau^{\text{Ind}}(U)\right] = \int \tau^{\text{Ind}}(u) f(u)\mathrm{d}u.
$$

Thus, even if the individual-level Kendall τ is zero for every u, the population-level Kendall τ may be nonzero. Usually, the population-level Kendall τ has a higher magnitude than the individual-level Kendall τ. However, theoretical analyses on the population-level Kendall τ and its relationship with the individual-level Kendall τ are less developed in the literature. A good starting point is to explore the expressions of the population-level Kendall τ under the joint frailty-copula model.

6.3   Validation of Surrogate Endpoints

Although the validation criteria for surrogate endpoints are still a subject of intense research, the current consensus is to base the validation on an approach of "correlation" based on a two-step method (Burzykowski et al. 2005; Rotolo et al. 2018). In the first step model and in order to assess the quality of the surrogate at the individual-level, they proposed to use a measure of association between the surrogate and the true endpoint using a copula model. In the second stage, a surrogate is termed as "valid" at trial-level if it is able to predict the effect of treatment on the true endpoint based on the observed effect of treatment on the surrogate endpoint. In order to make a formal validation process for survival endpoints, Burzykowski et al. (2001) proposed to use random effects models, where the quality of surrogate at the trial-level was assessed with a coefficient of determination (R^2). They proposed an adjusted trial-level surro-gacy measure, which takes estimation error of the treatment effects at the first step into account at the second stage. However, in each of their case studies, some convergence issues arise unless common baseline hazards across trials are assumed. Numerous articles have been published on the validation of surrogates, but the methods proposed are not suitable enough particularly in terms of identifiability or optimization (Burzykowski et al. 2005; Li et al. 2011). Renfro et al. (2012) described that convergence problems were frequently encountered in the first step (at individual-level). But even when the first step provides estimators, the second stage (at trial-level) does not always provide an estimate of the adjusted coefficients of determination (R^2). These numerical problems are frequently encountered and are influenced by the number and size of the trials as well as assumptions made on the baseline hazards among trials.

The FDA (the US Food and Drug Administration) adopts surrogate endpoints if they predict clinical outcome for the true endpoint. In many cancer studies, disease-free survival or progression-free survival is the surrogate endpoint for the true endpoint, namely OS. Rupp and Zuckerman (2017) reported that 18 anticancer drugs approved by the FDA on the basis of surrogate endpoints actually did not improve OS for patients. The reason behind this erroneous decision is difficult to identify. However, we should explore whether the problem comes from statistical tools.

In this context, it seems necessary to improve the existing methods to evaluate surrogate endpoints. It would be interesting to explore whether surrogate endpoints can be better validated by new statistical methods such as Rotolo et al. (2017). Also, the joint frailty-copula model (Chap. 3) is a tailored model to analyze the individual-level dependence via copulas in meta-analytic settings. However, developing a formal validation process of surrogacy requires further extensions of the joint frailty-copula model to incorporate the trial-level dependence. We are currently working on this topic.

6.4   Left Truncation

Left truncation often occurs if the timescale of endpoints is measured in terms of age. If the endpoint of interest is age at death, left truncation time corresponds to age at entry (entry age is not treated as a covariate). In other words, the endpoint is time to death measured from birth.

All the examples discussed in this book were concerned about the endpoints measured from the study entry time, so the problem of left truncation did not occur. Left truncation is particularly relevant for survival data arising from epidemiological and observational studies, where researchers cannot specify the valid study entry time. From a methodological point of view, there is a growing interest in the issue of left truncation arising from clustered survival data (Rondeau et al. 2017; Rodríguez-Girondo et al. 2018).

Left truncation yields a biased sampling since the patients are available only when the age at event exceeds the age at entry. All patients who have experienced the event before the entry are not sampled. In the survival analysis of a single endpoint, the bias due to left truncation can be adjusted by multiplying an inverse sampling probability to the likelihood function (Klein and Moeschberger 2003). In the analysis of two endpoints or clustered survival times, however, this adjustment is not always trivial. So far, there are three different approaches, called "naive", "updated", and "weighted approach" (Rodríguez-Girondo et al. 2018). Some method for handling left truncation was already suggested for the joint frailty-copula model (Rondeau et al. 2015; Emura et al. 2017) without numerical studies. More thorough analyses, like Rodríguez-Girondo et al. (2018), would be needed.

An interesting but challenging issue is to account for *dependent* left truncation. Traditional analyses for left-truncated survival data rely on *independent truncation* assumption (p. 126 of Klein and Moeschberger 2003). For instance, in the survival analysis of elderly residents, the age at entry to a retirement center is assumed to be independent of age at death (Hyde 1980). Several different tests for checking the assumption of independent truncation were developed (Emura and Wang 2010; Chiou et al. 2018). The effect of dependent truncation in competing risks analysis was studied by Bakoyannis and Touloumi (2017). To fit survival data with dependent left truncation, a copula model between event time and left truncation time has been considered (Chaieb et al. 2006; Emura and Wang 2012; Emura and Murotani 2015; Emura and Pan 2017). However, these methods cannot be directly applied to the case where two event times are subject to dependent truncation. In this case, one may consider two copulas, one for modeling dependent truncation and the other for modeling dependence between two event times.

6.5 Interactions

The models discussed in this book do not consider interactions between covariates. However, there are a few different cases, where interactions are of interest.

6.5.1 (Gene × Gene) Interaction

The (gene × gene) interaction may exist between those genes working in the same pathway. A two-stage analysis may be a simple way to discover such interactions, where the first stage considers main effects and the second stage considers their interactions. In the first stage, a univariate feature selection method is performed to select genes associated with survival (Chap. 4). In the second stage, for all pair of selected genes, one can perform an additional feature selection method as an attempt to discover interactions between the genes A variety of different methods could be considered in the second stage.

However, in our experience of adding interaction terms into a compound covariate predictor, there is only a modest improvement in prediction power. This might be because the main effects carry the majority of predictive information of survival, or the compound covariate implicitly incorporates some amount of interaction. There is an opportunity to apply a more sophisticated method that systematically incorporates the pathway or network information, such as those proposed by Kim et al. (2018), Wang and Chen (2018) and Choi et al. (2018). Exploration of the (gene × gene) interactions may not only improve prediction performance, but also lead to interesting insight about the biological mechanisms on the genes such as pathway structures.

6.5.2   (Gene × Time) Interaction

Time-varying effects of genetic covariates are another interesting issue to be investigated. If clinical follow-up of patients is long, the prognostic effect of genes may vary over time.

One may introduce time-varying effects of genes in the model by adding (gene × time) interaction terms. Specifically, the interaction term can be defined as CC × $f(t)$, where CC is a compound covariate (a linear combination of gene expressions) and $f(t)$ is a time function flexibly chosen by users. For instance, one can use $f(t) = \log(t + 1)$ (van Houwelingen and Putter 2011). In this way, the compound covariate accounts for "common" time-varying effects of genes. This approach would be effective if the majority of genes in the compound covariate share a similar time-varying effect on survival.

If the time-varying effects of individual genes are heterogeneous, one may categorize genes into subgroups. For instance, one can consider two subgroups, where genes of short-term effects and genes of long-term effects are separated. In this way, time-varying effects can be more homogeneous within the group. However, this strategy requires a way of grouping genes in order to reduce the heterogeneity of time-varying effects within a group.

Although one can straightforwardly define the joint frailty-copula model with time-varying effects, one cannot exploit the computational advantage of the spline models for the baseline hazard functions (i.e., the spline-based hazard functions have explicit integral formulas). As a result, likelihood-based inference becomes computationally demanding since the likelihood may involve some numerical integrations. One possible alternative is to impose piecewise exponential models for the baseline hazard functions. Some recent work on piecewise exponential models with copulas is referred to Emura and Michimae (2017).

6.6   Parametric Failure Time Models

Throughout this book, we focus on the spline-based model to fit the distributions of two endpoints. In this section, we shall briefly discuss the possibility of applying parametric models for analyzing correlated endpoints. Parametric models are usually simpler to use, interpret, and fit than semi-parametric models. However, as argued in Chap. 2, semi-parametric models are more frequently used in cancer research. One reason is that the hazard function for cancer patients rarely shows any simple pattern (e.g., monotonically increasing or decreasing), due to the complex processes of treatment regimens and their effects on patients. On the other hand, the hazard function of machines or items may exhibit simpler patterns as long as they are used in normal conditions. That is why parametric models are widely used in reliability analysis of manufactured items.

The Weibull distribution is one of the most frequently used parametric models in copula-based analysis for two endpoints. Escarela and Carrière (2003) proposed to fit a copula-based parametric model to competing risks data, where they used a copula for dependence between competing event times that follows the Weibull model. Burzykowski et al. (2001, 2005) proposed a bivariate Weibull model for jointly performing Cox regression for two endpoints with meta-analytic data; their method is implemented in an R package (Rotolo et al. 2018).

It is possible to apply the Weibull model to the joint frailty-copula model (Chap. 3; Emura et al. 2017) and to the dynamic prediction formulas (Chap. 5; Emura et al. 2018). Some advantages of the Weibull model is that one can compute the mean survival time, the correlation coefficient between endpoints, mean residual lifetime, and other quantities. Notice that all these moment-based quantities are difficult to be computed in the spline-based model that leads to improper distributions for the endpoints. To simplify the computation of moments, it is interesting to apply a conjugate distribution (gamma distribution) for the Weibull distribution (Molenberghs et al. 2015). We also notice that the accuracy of the feature selection and compound covariate methods of Chap. 4 may be improved by employing parametric models.

6.7   Compound Covariate

Tukey's compound covariate method, as detailed in Chap. 4, is a simple method to predict survival based on high-dimensional covariates. The compound covariate predictor is an ensemble of univariate models of individual covariates, and hence, it is simpler than most of the other prediction methods that use the penalized multivariate Cox model, such as the ridge and Lasso methods. Nevertheless, the compound covariate predictor may exhibit a competitive performance with these multivariate methods (Emura et al. 2012, 2018, 2019; Zhao et al. 2014; Chap. 4). While there are a number of real data analyses and simulation analyses on the compound covariate method, the theoretical studies are very scarce in the literature.

The unique property of Tukey's compound covariate is that it ignores the correlations between genes. Suppose that two genes are strongly correlated and both of them are univariately associated with survival (P-value < 0.001). Hence, the two genes are included in a compound covariate predictor. If the two genes were refitted into a multivariate Cox model, a usual strategy is to remove one of them to avoid the multicollinearity issue. The same logic may apply to a large number of genes univariately associated with survival. The compound covariate predictor includes all them by ignoring their correlations (i.e., without going through a multivariate Cox model).

In linear discriminant analysis, it has been well recognized that a predictor that ignores the correlations between individual covariates often performs better than a predictor that tries to account for dependence. In particular, Dudoit et al. (2002) reported a remarkable gain in predictive/classification accuracy by ignoring correlations among high-dimensional gene expressions. Some theoretical accounts for this phenomenon are available (Bickel and Levina 2004). However, the theory behind compound covariate in survival models has not been explored in the literature.

Another unique property of compound covariate is its *additive* property. Compound covariate aggregates univariate predictors to construct a multigene predictor. This resembles the idea of *naïve Bayes* (Bickel and Levina 2004), *jackknife model-averaging* (Hansen and Racine 2012) or *boosting* (Hastie et al. 2009). Consequently, removing one univariate predictor from the multigene predictor does not change much the whole model. This property produces the robustness of the compound covariate predictor against the cutoff value for feature selection as discussed in Chap. 4. It is worth exploring the robustness and accuracy of the compound covariate method through the aforementioned machine learning approaches.

References

Bakoyannis G, Touloumi G (2017) Impact of dependent left truncation in semiparametric competing risks methods: a simulation study. Commun Stat Simul Comput 46(3):2025–2042

Bickel PJ, Levina E (2004) Some theory for Fisher's linear discriminant function, naive Bayes, and some alternatives when there are many more variables than observations. Bernoulli 10(6):989–1010

Burzykowski T, Molenberghs G, Buyse M (eds) (2005) The evaluation of surrogate endpoints. Springer, New York

Burzykowski T, Molenberghs G, Buyse M, Geys H, Renard D (2001) Validation of surrogate end points in multiple randomized clinical trials with failure time end points. Appl Stat 50(4):405–422

Chaieb LL, Rivest LP, Abdous B (2006) Estimating survival under a dependent truncation. Biometrika 93(3):655–669

Chiou SH, Qian J, Mormino E et al (2018) Permutation tests for general dependent truncation. Comput Stat Data Anal 128:308–324

Choi J, Oh I, Seo S, Ahn J (2018) G2Vec: Distributed gene representations for identification of cancer prognostic genes. Sci Rep 8(1):13729

Dudoit S, Fridlyand J, Speed TP (2002) Comparison of discrimination methods for the classification of tumors using gene expression data. J Am Stat Assoc 97(457):77–87

Emura T, Chen YH, Chen HY (2012) Survival prediction based on compound covariate under Cox proportional hazard models. PLoS ONE 7(10):e47627. https://doi.org/10.1371/journal.pone.0047627

Emura T, Matsui S, Chen HY (2019) compound.Cox: univariate feature selection and compound covariate for predicting survival. Comput Methods Programs Biomed 168:21–37

Emura T, Michimae H (2017) A copula-based inference to piecewise exponential models under dependent censoring, with application to time to metamorphosis of salamander larvae. Environ Ecol Stat 24(1):151–173

Emura T, Murotani K (2015) An algorithm for estimating survival under a copula-based dependent truncation model. TEST 24(4):734–751

Emura T, Nakatochi M, Murotani K, Rondeau V (2017) A joint frailty-copula model between tumour progression and death for meta-analysis. Stat Methods Med Res 26(6):2649–2666

Emura T, Nakatochi M, Matsui S, Michimae H, Rondeau V (2018) Personalized dynamic prediction of death according to tumour progression and high-dimensional genetic factors: meta-analysis with a joint model. Stat Methods Med Res 27(9):2842–2858

Emura T, Pan CH (2017) Parametric likelihood inference and goodness-of-fit for dependently left-truncated data, a copula-based approach, Stat Pap. https://doi.org/10.1007/s00362-017-0947-z

Emura T, Wang W (2010) Testing quasi-independence for truncation data. J Multivar Anal 101:223–239

Emura T, Wang W (2012) Nonparametric maximum likelihood estimation for dependent truncation data based on copulas. J Multivar Anal 110:171–188

Escarela G, Carrière JF (2003) Fitting competing risks with an assumed copula. Statist Methods Med Res 12(4):333–349

González JR, Fernandez E, Moreno V, Ribes J et al (2005) Sex differences in hospital readmission among colorectal cancer patients. J Epidemiol Community Health 59(6):506–511

Hansen BE, Racine JS (2012) Jackknife model averaging. J Econometrics 167(1):38–46

Hastie T, Tibshirani R, Friedman J (2009) The elements of statistical learning. Springer, New York

Hyde J (1980) Survival analysis with incomplete observations. In: Miller RG, Efron B, Brown BW, Moses LE (eds) Biostatistics casebook. Wiley, New York, pp 31–46

Kim M, Oh I, Ahn J (2018) An improved method for prediction of cancer prognosis by network learning. Genes 9:478

Klein JP, Moeschberger ML (2003) Survival analysis techniques for censored and truncated data. Springer, New York

Li Y, Taylor JM, Elliott MR, Sargent DJ (2011) Causal assessment of surrogacy in a meta-analysis of colorectal cancer trials. Biostatistics 12(3):478–492

Li Z, Chinchilli VM, Wang M (2019) A Bayesian joint model of recurrent events and a terminal event. Biometrical Journal 61(1):187–202

Molenberghs G, Verbeke G, Efendi A, Braekers R, Demétrio CG (2015) A combined gamma frailty and normal random-effects model for repeated, over dispersed time-to-event data. Stat Methods Med Res 24(4):434–452

Renfro LA, Shi Q, Sargent DJ, Carlin BP (2012) Bayesian adjusted R2 for the meta-analytic evaluation of surrogate time-to-event endpoints in clinical trials. Stat Med 31(8):743–761

Rodríguez-Girondo M, Deelen J, Slagboom EP, Houwing-Duistermaat JJ (2018) Survival analysis with delayed entry in selected families with application to human longevity. Stat Methods Med Res 27(3):933–954

Rondeau V, Gonzalez JR (2005) frailtypack: a computer program for the analysis of correlated failure time data using penalized likelihood estimation. Comput Methods Programs Biomed 80(2):154–164

Rondeau V, Mauguen A, Laurent A, Berr C, Helmer C (2017) Dynamic prediction models for clustered and interval-censored outcomes: investigating the intra-couple correlation in the risk of dementia. Stat Methods Med Res 26(5):2168–2183

Rondeau V, Pignon JP, Michiels S (2015) A joint model for dependence between clustered times to tumour progression and deaths: a meta-analysis of chemotherapy in head and neck cancer. Stat Methods Med Res 24(6):711–729

Rotolo F, Paoletti X, Burzykowski T, Buyse M, Michiels S (2017) Poisson approach to the validation of failure time surrogate endpoints in individual patient data meta-analyses, Stat Methods Med Res. https://doi.org/10.1177/0962280217718582

Rotolo F, Paoletti X. Michiels S (2018). surrosurv: An R package for the evaluation of failure time surrogate endpoints in individual patient data meta-analyses of randomized clinical trials. Comput Methods Programs Biomed 155: 189–198

Rupp T, Zuckerman D (2017) Quality of life, overall survival, and costs of cancer drugs approved based on surrogate endpoints. JAMA Internal Medicine 177(2):276–277

van Houwelingen HC, Putter H (2011) Dynamic prediction in clinical survival analysis. CRC Press, New York

Wang JH, Chen YH (2018) Overlapping group screening for detection of gene-gene interactions: application to gene expression profiles with survival trait. BMC Bioinformatics 201819:335

Zhao SD, Parmigiani G, Huttenhower C, Waldron L (2014) Más-o-menos: a simple sign averaging method for discrimination in genomic data analysis. Bioinformatics 30(21):3062–3069

Appendix A
Spline Basis Functions

This appendix defines the spline basis functions used in $\lambda_0(t) = \sum_{\ell=1}^{5} h_\ell M_\ell(t) = \mathbf{h}'\mathbf{M}(t)$. We also calculate the roughness $\int \ddot{\lambda}_0(t)^2 dt$.

For a knot sequence $\xi_1 < \xi_2 < \xi_3$ with an equally spaced mesh $\Delta = \xi_2 - \xi_1 = \xi_3 - \xi_2$, let $z_i(t) = (t - \xi_i)/\Delta$ for $i = 1, 2,$ and 3. Define *M-spline basis* functions as

$$M_1(t) = -\frac{4\mathbf{I}(\xi_1 \leq t < \xi_2)}{\Delta} z_2(t)^3, \quad M_5(t) = \frac{4\mathbf{I}(\xi_2 \leq t < \xi_3)}{\Delta} z_2(t)^3,$$

$$M_2(t) = \frac{\mathbf{I}(\xi_1 \leq t < \xi_2)}{2\Delta}\{7z_1(t)^3 - 18z_1(t)^2 + 12z_1(t)\} - \frac{\mathbf{I}(\xi_2 \leq t < \xi_3)}{2\Delta} z_3(t)^3,$$

$$M_3(t) = \frac{\mathbf{I}(\xi_1 \leq t < \xi_2)}{\Delta}\{-2z_1(t)^3 + 3z_1(t)^2\} + \frac{\mathbf{I}(\xi_2 \leq t < \xi_3)}{\Delta}\{2z_2(t)^3 - 3z_2(t)^2 + 1\},$$

$$M_4(t) = \frac{\mathbf{I}(\xi_1 \leq t < \xi_2)}{2\Delta} z_1(t)^3 + \frac{\mathbf{I}(\xi_2 \leq t < \xi_3)}{2\Delta}\{-7z_2(t)^3 + 3z_2(t)^2 + 3z_2(t) + 1\}.$$

Define the *I-spline basis* function, $I_\ell(t) = \int_{\xi_1}^{t} M_\ell(u) du$, which can be written as

$$I_1(t) = 1 - z_2(t)^4 \mathbf{I}(\xi_1 \leq t < \xi_2), \quad I_5(t) = z_2(t)^4 \mathbf{I}(\xi_2 \leq t < \xi_3),$$

$$I_2(t) = \{\frac{7}{8} z_1(t)^4 - 3z_1(t)^3 + 3z_1(t)^2\}\mathbf{I}(\xi_1 \leq t < \xi_2) + \{1 - \frac{1}{8} z_3(t)^4\}\mathbf{I}(\xi_2 \leq t < \xi_3),$$

$$I_3(t) = \{-\frac{1}{2} z_1(t)^4 + z_1(t)^3\}\mathbf{I}(\xi_1 \leq t < \xi_2) + \{\frac{1}{2} + \frac{1}{2} z_2(t)^4 - z_2(t)^3 + z_2(t)\}\mathbf{I}(\xi_2 \leq t < \xi_3),$$

$$I_4(t) = \frac{1}{8} z_1(t)^4 \mathbf{I}(\xi_1 \leq t < \xi_2) + \{\frac{1}{8} - \frac{7}{8} z_2(t)^4 + \frac{1}{2} z_2(t)^3 + \frac{3}{4} z_2(t)^2 + \frac{1}{2} z_2(t)\}\mathbf{I}(\xi_2 \leq t < \xi_3).$$

© The Author(s), under exclusive license to Springer Nature Singapore Pte Ltd. 2019

T. Emura et al., *Survival Analysis with Correlated Endpoints*, JSS Research Series in Statistics, https://doi.org/10.1007/978-981-13-3516-7

The second derivatives of the M-spline basis functions are

$$
\ddot{M}_1(t) = -\frac{24}{\Delta^3} z_2(t) \mathbf{I}(\xi_1 \le t < \xi_2), \quad \ddot{M}_5(t) = \frac{24}{\Delta^3} z_2(t) \mathbf{I}(\xi_2 \le t < \xi_3),
$$

$$
\ddot{M}_2(t) = \left\{ \frac{21}{\Delta^3} z_1(t) - \frac{18}{\Delta^3} \right\} \mathbf{I}(\xi_1 \le t < \xi_2) - \frac{3}{\Delta^3} z_3(t) \mathbf{I}(\xi_2 \le t < \xi_3),
$$

$$
\ddot{M}_3(t) = \left\{ -\frac{12}{\Delta^3} z_1(t) + \frac{6}{\Delta^3} \right\} \mathbf{I}(\xi_1 \le t < \xi_2) + \left\{ \frac{12}{\Delta^3} z_2(t) - \frac{6}{\Delta^3} \right\} \mathbf{I}(\xi_2 \le t < \xi_3),
$$

$$
\ddot{M}_4(t) = \frac{3}{\Delta^3} z_1(t) \mathbf{I}(\xi_1 \le t < \xi_2) + \left\{ -\frac{21}{\Delta^3} z_2(t) + \frac{3}{\Delta^3} \right\} \mathbf{I}(\xi_2 \le t < \xi_3).
$$

It follows that

$$
\int \ddot{M}_1(t)^2 dt = \frac{192}{\Delta^5}, \int \ddot{M}_2(t)^2 dt = \frac{96}{\Delta^5}, \int \ddot{M}_3(t)^2 dt = \frac{24}{\Delta^5}, \int \ddot{M}_4(t)^2 dt = \frac{96}{\Delta^5}, \int \ddot{M}_5(t)^2 dt = \frac{192}{\Delta^5},
$$

$$
\int \ddot{M}_1(t)\ddot{M}_2(t) dt = -\frac{132}{\Delta^5}, \int \ddot{M}_1(t)\ddot{M}_3(t) dt = \frac{24}{\Delta^5}, \int \ddot{M}_1(t)\ddot{M}_4(t) dt = \frac{12}{\Delta^5}, \int \ddot{M}_1(t)\ddot{M}_5(t) dt = 0,
$$

$$
\int \ddot{M}_2(t)\ddot{M}_3(t) dt = -\frac{24}{\Delta^5}, \int \ddot{M}_2(t)\ddot{M}_4(t) dt = -\frac{12}{\Delta^5}, \int \ddot{M}_2(t)\ddot{M}_5(t) dt = \frac{12}{\Delta^5},
$$

$$
\int \ddot{M}_3(t)\ddot{M}_4(t) dt = -\frac{24}{\Delta^5}, \int \ddot{M}_3(t)\ddot{M}_5(t) dt = \frac{24}{\Delta^5}, \int \ddot{M}_4(t)\ddot{M}_5(t) dt = -\frac{132}{\Delta^5},
$$

where the range of integral is $(\xi_1, \xi_3]$. Then, the penalization term is explicitly computed as

$$
\int \ddot{\lambda}_0(t)^2 dt = \sum_{k=1}^{5} \sum_{\ell=1}^{5} h_k h_\ell \int \ddot{M}_k(t)\ddot{M}_\ell(t) dt
$$

$$
= \frac{1}{\Delta^5} \mathbf{h}' \begin{bmatrix} 192 & -132 & 24 & 12 & 0 \\ -132 & 96 & -24 & -12 & 12 \\ 24 & -24 & 24 & -24 & 24 \\ 12 & -12 & -24 & 96 & -132 \\ 0 & 12 & 24 & -132 & 192 \end{bmatrix} \mathbf{h} = \mathbf{h}' \Omega \mathbf{h}.
$$

All the expressions mentioned above were derived in the supplementary material of Emura et al. (2017). The computational programs of the M- and I-spline basis functions are available in the *joint.Cox* R package (Emura 2019). These basis functions were derived from the general definition of M-spline basis functions given by Ramsay (1988). The derivations of these basis functions are detailed in Appendix A of Emura and Chen (2018).

References

Emura T (2019) joint.Cox: joint frailty-copula models for tumour progression and death in meta-analysis. CRAN.

Emura T, Chen YH (2018) Analysis of survival data with dependent censoring, copula-based approaches. JSS Research Series in Statistics. Springer.

Emura T, Nakatochi M, Murotani K, Rondeau V (2017) A joint frailty-copula model between tumour progression and death for meta-analysis. Stat Methods Med Res 26(6):2649–2666

Ramsay J (1988) Monotone regression spline in action. Stat Sci 3:425–461

Appendix B
R Codes for the Ovarian Cancer Data Analysis

B1. Using the *CXCL12* Gene as a Covariate

```
library(joint.Cox)
data(dataOvarian)
t.event=dataOvarian$t.event  ## time-to-relapse (TTP) ##
event=dataOvarian$event  ## indicator for relapse ##
t.death=dataOvarian$t.death  ## time-to-death (OS) ##
death=dataOvarian$death  ## indicator for death ##
Z1=dataOvarian$CXCL12  ## gene expression of CXCL12 ##
group=dataOvarian$group  ## study indicator (4 studies) ##
alpha_given=0
grid=seq(10, 1e+17, length=30)  ## grid for searching the best smoothing parameter ##
set.seed(1)
res=jointCox.reg(t.event=t.event, event=event, t.death=t.death, death=death,
                 Z1=Z1, Z2=Z1, group=group, alpha=alpha_given,
                 kappa1=grid, kappa2=grid, LCV.plot=TRUE, Adj=500)
res

#### Plot the baseline hazard function for TTP ####
par( mfrow=c(1, 1) )
t_min=min(t.event)  ## lower bound for the baseline hazard function
t_max=max(t.death)  ## upper bound for the baseline hazard function

r1_func=function(t){ as.numeric( M.spline (t, t_min, t_max)%*%(res$g) ) }
```

© The Author(s), under exclusive license to Springer Nature Singapore Pte Ltd. 2019   109
T. Emura et al., *Survival Analysis with Correlated Endpoints*,
JSS Research Series in Statistics, https://doi.org/10.1007/978-981-13-3516-7

```r
r1_Low_func=function(t){ ## lower confidence limit
 M_vec=M.spline (t, t_min, t_max)
 r1_V=M_vec%*%(res$g_var)%*%t(M_vec)
 as.numeric( M_vec%*%(res$g)-1.96*sqrt(diag(r1_V)) )
}

r1_Up_func=function(t){ ## upper confidence limit
    M_vec=M.spline (t, t_min, t_max)
    r1_V=M_vec%*%(res$g_var)%*%t(M_vec)
    as.numeric( M_vec%*%(res$g)+1.96*sqrt(diag(r1_V)) )
}

curve( r1_func, t_min, t_max, lwd=3, xlab="Days",
        ylab="Baseline hazard", ylim=c(0.00003, 0.0012), xlim=c(0, 5500) )
curve(r1_Low_func, t_min, t_max, lty="dotted", add=TRUE, col="blue")
curve(r1_Up_func, t_min, t_max, lty="dotted", add=TRUE, col="blue")
AA=c("Hazard function for TTP","95% CI")
BB=c("solid", "dotted")
CC=c("black", "blue")
legend(1800, 0.0011, AA, lwd=c(3, 1), merge = TRUE, lty=BB, col=CC)

#### Plot the baseline hazard function for OS ####
r2_func=function(t){as.numeric( M.spline (t, t_min, t_max)%*%(res$h) )}

r2_Low_func=function(t){ ## lower confidence limit
 r2_V=M.spline (t, t_min, t_max)%*%(res$h_var)%*%t(M.spline (t, t_min, t_max))
 as.numeric( M.spline (t,t_min, t_max)%*%(res$h)-1.96*sqrt(diag(r2_V)) )
}
r2_Up_func=function(t) { ## upper confidence limit
 r2_V=M.spline (t, t_min, t_max)%*%(res$h_var)%*%t(M.spline (t, t_min, t_max))
 as.numeric( M.spline (t, t_min, t_max)%*%(res$h)+1.96*sqrt(diag(r2_V)) )
}

curve(r2_func, t_min, t_max,lwd=3, lty="dotdash",xlab="Days",add=TRUE)
curve(r2_Low_func, t_min, t_max, lty="dotted",lwd=1,add=TRUE,col="red")
curve(r2_Up_func, t_min, t_max, lty="dotted",lwd=1,add=TRUE,col="red")

AA=c("Hazard function for OS", "95% CI")
BB=c("dotdash", "dotted")
CC=c("black", "red")
legend(3800, 0.0008, AA, lwd=c(3,1), merge = TRUE, lty=BB, col=CC)

########## Relative risk (RR) ##############
RR_TTP=c(RR=exp(res$beta1[1]), Low=exp(res$beta1[1]-1.96*res$beta1[2]),
            Up=exp(res$beta1[1]+1.96*res$beta1[2]))
RR_OS=c(RR=exp(res$beta2[1]), Low=exp(res$beta2[1]-1.96*res$beta2[2]),
            Up=exp(res$beta2[1]+1.96*res$beta2[2]))

list(alpha=alpha_given,
    RR1=round(RR_TTP,2), RR2=round(RR_OS,2), eta=round(res$eta,4),
    theta=round(res$theta,4), tau=round(res$tau,4)
)
```

B2. Using the Compound Covariates (CCs) and Residual Tumour as Covariates

```
library(joint.Cox)
library(compound.Cox)

data(dataOvarian1)
data(dataOvarian2)
t.event=dataOvarian1$t.event   ## time-to-relapse (TTP) ##
event=dataOvarian1$event   ## indicator for relapse ##
t.death=dataOvarian2$t.death   ## time-to-death (OS) ##
death=dataOvarian2$death   ## indicator for death ##
residual=dataOvarian1[,4]   ## residual tumour size (>=1cm vs. <1cm)
group=dataOvarian1[,3]   ## study indicator (4 studies) ##
X.mat1=dataOvarian1[,-c(1,2,3,4)]   ### genes associated with TTP
X.mat2=dataOvarian2[,-c(1,2,3,4)]   ## genes associated with OS
Symbol1=colnames(dataOvarian1)[-c(1,2,3,4)]   ## gene symbols for TTP
Symbol2=colnames(dataOvarian2)[-c(1,2,3,4)]   ## gene symbols for OS
X.mat1=as.matrix(X.mat1)
X.mat2=as.matrix(X.mat2)
q1=ncol(X.mat1) ## the number of genes associated with TTP ##
q2=ncol(X.mat2) ## the number of genes associated with OS ##


##### Compound covariate for TTP ####
res=uni.Wald(t.event,event,X.mat1)
coef1=res$beta
data.frame( gene=names(res$beta)[order(res$P)], P=res$P[order(res$P)],
        coef=round(coef1[order(res$P)],3) )
CC1_train=X.mat1%*%coef1 ### Compound covariate for TTP ###
mu1=mean(CC1_train)
sigma1=sd(CC1_train)
round(c(mu1=mu1,sigma1=sigma1),3)


##### Compound covariate for OS ####
res=uni.Wald(t.death,death,X.mat2)
coef2=res$beta
data.frame( gene=names(res$beta)[order(res$P)], P=res$P[order(res$P)],
        coef=round(coef2[order(res$P)],3) )
CC2_train=X.mat2%*%coef2 ### Compound covariate for OS ###
mu2=mean(CC2_train)
sigma2=sd(CC2_train)
round(c(mu2=mu2,sigma2=sigma2),3)


mu2+2*sigma2  ## high-risk
mu2-2*sigma2  ## low-risk


############## Fit the joint frailty-copula model ################
grid=c(seq(10,1e+17,length=100))
set.seed(1)
res=jointCox.reg(t.event=t.event, event=event, t.death=t.death, death=death,
        Z1=(CC1_train-mu1)/sigma1, Z2=cbind( residual,(CC2_train-mu2)/sigma2 ),
        group=group, alpha=0, convergence.par = TRUE,
        kappa1=grid, kappa2=grid, LCV.plot=TRUE, Randomize_num=1)

########## Relative risk #########
```

```
RR_gamma1=exp(res$beta1[c(1,3,4)])
RR_beta2=exp(res$beta2[c(1,5,7)])
RR_gamma2=exp(res$beta2[c(2,6,8)])

########## Summarize estimates #############
list(RR_gamma1=round(RR_gamma1,2),RR_beta2=round(RR_beta2,2),
   RR_gamma2=round(RR_gamma2,2),eta=round(res$eta,2),
   theta=round(res$theta,1),tau=round(res$tau,2))

list(gamma1=round(res$beta1,3),beta2=round(res$beta2[c(1,3,5,7)],3),
   gamma2=round(res$beta2[c(2,4,6,8)],3),eta=round(res$eta,3),
   theta=round(res$theta,2),tau=round(res$tau,2),
   g=round(res$g,2),h=round(res$h,2)
)
```

The codes do not include the calculations for the patient-level survival curves and their CIs.

Appendix C
Derivation of Prediction Formulas

Case I: Given that the patient does not experience tumour progression before time t (i.e., $X > t$), the conditional failure function is

$$
\begin{aligned}
F(t, t+w \mid X > t, \mathbf{Z}) &= \Pr(D \leq t+w \mid D > t, X > t, \mathbf{Z}) \\
&= \frac{\Pr(D > t, X > t \mid \mathbf{Z}) - \Pr(D > t+w, X > t \mid \mathbf{Z})}{\Pr(D > t, X > t \mid \mathbf{Z})} \\
&= \frac{\int_0^\infty (\Pr(D > t, X > t \mid u, \mathbf{Z}) - \Pr(D > t+w, X > t \mid u, \mathbf{Z})) f_\eta(u) du}{\int_0^\infty \Pr(D > t, X > t \mid u, \mathbf{Z}) f_\eta(u) du} \\
&= \frac{\int_0^\infty (C_\theta[S_X(t \mid u), S_D(t \mid u)] - C_\theta[S_X(t \mid u), S_D(t+w \mid u)]) f_\eta(u) du}{\int_0^\infty C_\theta[S_X(t \mid u), S_D(t \mid u)] f_\eta(u) du},
\end{aligned}
$$

and the conditional hazard function is

$$
\begin{aligned}
\lambda(t \mid X > t, \mathbf{Z}, u) &= \Pr(t < D \leq t+dt \mid X > t, D > t, \mathbf{Z}, u)/dt \\
&= \frac{\Pr(X > t, t < D \leq t+dt \mid \mathbf{Z}, u)}{dt \cdot \Pr(X > t, D > t \mid \mathbf{Z}, u)} \\
&= -\frac{\Pr(X > t, D > t+dt \mid \mathbf{Z}, u) - \Pr(X > t, D > t \mid \mathbf{Z}, u)}{dt \cdot \Pr(X > t, D > t \mid \mathbf{Z}, u)} \\
&= \frac{-\partial \Pr(X > t, D > y \mid \mathbf{Z}, u)/\partial y \big|_{y=t}}{\Pr(X > t, D > t \mid \mathbf{Z}, u)} \\
&= \{-\partial S_D(t \mid u)/\partial t\} \frac{C_\theta^{[0,1]}[S_X(t \mid u), S_D(t \mid u)]}{C_\theta[S_X(t \mid u), S_D(t \mid u)]} \\
&= \lambda_D(t \mid u) \frac{S_D(t \mid u) C_\theta^{[0,1]}[S_X(t \mid u), S_D(t \mid u)]}{C_\theta[S_X(t \mid u), S_D(t \mid u)]}.
\end{aligned}
$$

© The Author(s), under exclusive license to Springer Nature Singapore Pte Ltd. 2019
T. Emura et al., *Survival Analysis with Correlated Endpoints*,
JSS Research Series in Statistics, https://doi.org/10.1007/978-981-13-3516-7

Case II: Given that the patient experiences tumour progression at time $x \leq t$, the conditional failure function is

$$
\begin{aligned}
F(t, t+w \mid X = x, \mathbf{Z}) &= \Pr(D \leq t+w \mid D > t, X = x, \mathbf{Z}) \\
&= \frac{\Pr(D > t, X = x \mid \mathbf{Z}) - \Pr(D > t+w, X = x \mid \mathbf{Z})}{\Pr(D > t, X = x \mid \mathbf{Z})} \\
&= \frac{\int_0^\infty \Pr((D > t, X = x \mid u, \mathbf{Z}) - \Pr(D > t+w, X = x \mid u, \mathbf{Z})) f_\eta(u) \mathrm{d}u}{\int_0^\infty \Pr(D > t, X = x \mid u, \mathbf{Z}) f_\eta(u) \mathrm{d}u} \\
&= \frac{\int_0^\infty \left(-\frac{\partial}{\partial x} \Pr(D > t, X > x \mid u, \mathbf{Z}) - \left\{ -\frac{\partial}{\partial x} \Pr(D > t+w, X > x \mid u, \mathbf{Z}) f_\eta(u) \mathrm{d}u \right\} \right)}{\int_0^\infty -\frac{\partial}{\partial x} \Pr(D > t, X > x \mid u, \mathbf{Z}) f_\eta(u) \mathrm{d}u} \\
&= \frac{\int_0^\infty \left(-\frac{\partial}{\partial x} C_\theta[S_X(x|u), S_D(t|u)] - \left\{ -\frac{\partial}{\partial x} C_\theta[S_X(x|u), S_D(t+w|u)] \right\} \right) f_\eta(u) \mathrm{d}u}{\int_0^\infty -\frac{\partial}{\partial x} C_\theta[S_X(x|u), S_D(t|u)] f_\eta(u) \mathrm{d}u} \\
&= \frac{\int_0^\infty \left(C_\theta^{[1,0]}[S_X(x|u), S_D(t|u)] - C_\theta^{[1,0]}[S_X(x|u), S_D(t+w|u)] \right) \lambda_X(x|u) S_X(x|u) f_\eta(u) \mathrm{d}u}{\int_0^\infty C_\theta^{[1,0]}[S_X(x|u), S_D(t|u)] \lambda_X(x|u) S_X(x|u) f_\eta(u) \mathrm{d}u},
\end{aligned}
$$

and the conditional hazard function is

$$
\begin{aligned}
\lambda(t \mid X = x, \mathbf{Z}, u) &= \Pr(t < D \leq t+dt \mid X = x, D > t, \mathbf{Z}, u)/\mathrm{d}t \\
&= \frac{\Pr(X = x, t < D \leq t+dt \mid \mathbf{Z}, u)}{\mathrm{d}t \cdot \Pr(X = x, D > t \mid \mathbf{Z}, u)} \\
&= -\frac{\Pr(X = x, D > t+dt \mid \mathbf{Z}, u) - \Pr(X = x, D > t \mid \mathbf{Z}, u)}{\mathrm{d}t \cdot \Pr(X = x, D > t \mid \mathbf{Z}, u)} \\
&= -\frac{\partial \Pr(X = x, D > t \mid \mathbf{Z}, u)/\partial t}{\Pr(X = x, D > t \mid \mathbf{Z}, u)} \\
&= -\frac{\partial^2 \Pr(X > x, D > t \mid \mathbf{Z}, u)/\partial x \partial t}{\partial \Pr(X > x, D > t \mid \mathbf{Z}, u)/\partial x} \\
&= -\frac{\partial S_D(t|u)}{\partial t} \frac{C_\theta^{[1,1]}[S_X(x|u), S_D(t|u)]}{C_\theta^{[1,0]}[S_X(x|u), S_D(t|u)]} \\
&= \lambda_D(t|u) \frac{S_D(t|u) C_\theta^{[1,1]}[S_X(x|u), S_D(t|u)]}{C_\theta^{[1,0]}[S_X(x|u), S_D(t|u)]}.
\end{aligned}
$$

If one applies the independence copula $C(v, w) = vw$ to the previous formulas,

$$F(t, t+w \mid X > t, \mathbf{Z}) = \frac{\int_0^\infty (S_D(t \mid u) - S_D(t + w \mid u)) S_X(t \mid u) f_\eta(u) du}{\int_0^\infty S_D(t \mid u) S_X(t \mid u) f_\eta(u) du},$$

$$F(t, t+w \mid X = x, \mathbf{Z}) = \frac{\int_0^\infty (S_D(t \mid u) - S_D(t + w \mid u)) \lambda_X(x \mid u) S_X(x \mid u) f_\eta(u) du}{\int_0^\infty S_D(t \mid u) \lambda_X(x \mid u) S_X(x \mid u) f_\eta(u) du},$$

$$\lambda(t \mid X > t, \mathbf{Z}, u) = \lambda(t \mid X = x, \mathbf{Z}, u) = \lambda_D(t \mid u).$$

Index

© The Author(s), under exclusive license to Springer Nature Singapore Pte Ltd. 2019   117
T. Emura et al., *Survival Analysis with Correlated Endpoints*,
JSS Research Series in Statistics, https://doi.org/10.1007/978-981-13-3516-7

Printed in the United States
By Bookmasters